Delivery of Health Care in Urban Underserved Areas

Edited by
Salvinija G. Kernaghan

AMERICAN HOSPITAL ASSOCIATION
840 North Lake Shore Drive
Chicago, Illinois 60611

Library of Congress Cataloging in Publication Data

Main entry under title:

Delivery of health care in urban underserved areas.

   Report of a conference held in Washington, Feb. 13-14, 1978 which was sponsored by the American Hospital Association and the Hospital Research and Educational Trust.
   Bibliography: p.
   1. Medical care—United States—Congresses.
2. Medically underserved areas—United States—Congresses. 3. Urban health—United States—Congresses.
I. Kernaghan, Salinija G. II. American Hospital Association. III. Hospital Research and Educational Trust.
RA395.A3D44   362.1'0973   79-21168
ISBN 0-87258-278-7

AHA catalog no. 1165
©1979 by the
American Hospital Association
840 North Lake Shore Drive
Chicago, Illinois 60611

All rights reserved
Printed in the U.S.A.
3.5M-10/79-6826

Printed and designed by
Visual Images Inc.
Des Plaines, Illinois

Contents

Foreword v
Participants vii
Keynote Address 1
    Cost Control versus Public Welfare: The Illinois Experience . 3
    Keynote address by Richard H. Newhouse

Payment for Health Care 11
    The Role of Urban Hospitals in the Nation's
    Health Economy 13
    Overview presentation by Nora Piore

    Tight Money and Expanding Needs: Some Answers to
    these Urban Problems 26
    Summary of workshops

Delivery of Health Care 43
    Accessible and Acceptable: What Urban Health
    Care Is Not 45
    Overview presentation by Mamie C. Hughes

    Patient and Consumer Participation: Is It Always
    for the Better? 51
    Summary of workshops

Consumer Power and Medical Manpower 67
    Managing Manpower Shortages: How To Fill the Gaps 69
    Overview presentation by Haynes Rice

    The Manpower Training Establishment: Target of a
    Changing Value System 76
    Summary of workshops

Summary and Recommendations 95
    Some Familiar Exhortations 97

Selected Bibliography 105

Foreword

Because of the constantly increasing complexity of health care delivery in urban areas, especially underserved areas, the American Hospital Association and the Hospital Research and Educational Trust, with support from the McDonald's Corporation, conducted an invitational conference on the delivery of health care in urban underserved areas. The purpose of the conference was to provide a setting in which knowledgeable persons could develop and discuss the major issues in urban health care.

The conference, held in Washington, DC, on February 13-14, 1978, brought together representative urban providers and technical experts who work in this complex arena every day and congressional and federal agency staff members who promulgate legislation and regulations and fund programs that affect urban efforts.

For two days the participants worked together to discover their common concerns and air their differences. Sessions were held on urban resources, accessibility and acceptability of health care services, and manpower. An overview of each subject was presented, and the participants were then assigned to one of three workshops. The lively discussions that ensued were based on the information presented in the overviews. At the initiatives, which closed the conference, summaries of the workshop discussions became the basis for recommendations for future actions.

All the speeches and workshop discussions were recorded. However, because of the technical limitations of recording the workshops, it was not possible to identify each speaker by name.

Many persons were responsible for the success of the conference. They contributed advice, interest, and hard work, and their contributions are acknowledged with gratitude.

The conference was developed with the support of the Public-General Hospital Section of the American Hospital Association. The members of the planning committee were Stanley Bergen, M.D., pres ident, College of Medicine and Dentistry, Newark, NJ; Ruth M. Rothstein, president, Mount Sinai Hospital Medical Center of Chicago, and Bernard M. Weinstein, commissioner of hospitals, Westchester County Medical Center, Valhalla, NY.

This report was prepared by Salvinija G. Kernaghan, Chicago, from transcripts of the recordings. Editorial services were provided by Sandra L. Weiss, assistant editor, and Dorothy Saxner, manager, AHA's Department of Books and Newsletters.

Appreciation is expressed to the McDonald's Corporation for its financial assistance. Special thanks are extended to keynote speaker Richard H. Newhouse, Illinois state senator, and the speakers who provided the overviews for the conference discussions: Nora Piore, associate director and professor of health administration-economics, Columbia University Center for Community Health Systems, New York City; Mamie Hughes, vice-chairperson, County Legislature of Jackson County, Kansas City, MO; and Haynes Rice, administrator, Howard University Hospital, Washington, DC.

Deepest gratitude goes to the conference participants—the many health care providers, representatives of other national organizations, and federal officials from both the executive and legislative branches of government—who contributed their experience, knowledge, effort, and time to make the conference productive for those who participated and useful to the field.

Susanne Batko, Conference Coordinator
Assistant Director
Center for Urban Hospitals
American Hospital Association

Participants

SPEAKERS

Leo J. Gehrig, M.D.
Senior Vice-President
American Hospital Association
Washington, DC

Mamie Hughes
Vice-Chairperson
County Legislature of Jackson County
Kansas City, MO

Richard H. Newhouse
Illinois State Senate
24th Illinois Senatorial District

Nora Piore
Associate Director, Professor
 of Health Administration-Economics
Columbia University Center
 for Community Health Systems
New York, NY

Haynes Rice
Administrator
Howard University Hospital
Washington, DC

DISCUSSION LEADERS

Stanley Bergen, M.D.
President
College of Medicine and Dentistry
Newark, NJ

Clifton A. Cole
Executive Director
Watts Health Foundation, Inc.
Los Angeles, CA

Gordon M. Derzon
Superintendent
University of Wisconsin Hospitals
Madison, WI

Leonard D. Fenninger, M.D.
Group Vice-President for Medical Education
American Medical Association
Chicago, IL

Symond R. Gottlieb
Executive Director
Greater Detroit Area Hospital Council Inc.
Detroit, MI

Robert C. Gronbach
Director of Employee Relations and Assistant Director
Hartford Hospital
Hartford, CT

Arthur E. Hess
Director
Commission on Public-General Hospitals
Washington, DC

Gordon D. Howe
Deputy Manager for Operations and Finance
Denver General Hospital
Denver, CO

Donald Kummerfeld
Director
Emergency Financial Control Board
New York, NY

LeRoy P. Levitt, M.D.
Vice-President for Medical Affairs
Mount Sinai Hospital Medical Center
Chicago, IL

Maurice V. Russell, Ed.D.
Director, Social Services
New York University Medical Center
New York, NY

Bernard M. Weinstein
Commissioner of Hospitals
Westchester County Medical Center
Valhalla, NY

PARTICIPANTS

Frederic Abramson, Ph.D.
President
Health Management Systems
Laytonsville, MD

Mary Lou Anderson
Consultant
Office of Legislation (Health)
Office of the Secretary
Department of Health, Education, and Welfare
Washington, DC

Bertha D. Atelsek
Director
Division of Health Services Evaluation
National Center for Health Services Research
Health Resources Administration
Department of Health, Education, and Welfare
Rockville, MD

Melvin Bailey
Assistant to Sen. Richard Newhouse
Illinois State Senate
Chicago, IL

Susan Bailey
Congressional Research Service
Library of Congress
Washington, DC

James D. Bentley, Ph.D.
Assistant Director
Department of Teaching Hospitals
Association of American Medical Colleges
Washington, DC

Robert Berenson, M.D.
Domestic Policy Staff
Executive Office of the President
Washington, DC

C. Howard Bozeman
County Judge
Knox County
Knoxville, TN

Ray Brown
Director, Division of Long Term Care
Health Care Financing Administration
U.S. Public Health Service
Washington, DC

Participants

Anita W. Burney
Chief, Program Coordination Branch
Division of Hospitals and Clinics
U.S. Public Health Service
Washington, DC

Mary Cahill
Program Analyst
National Institute on Drug Abuse
U.S. Public Health Service
Washington, DC

Dave Callagy
Chief, Recruitment Services Branch
Division of Clinical Services
Bureau of Community Health Services
U.S. Public Health Service
Washington, DC

Leonard Cohen
Legislative Service Branch
Bureau of Community Health Services
U.S. Public Health Service
Washington, DC

George A. Courie
Special Assistant to the Director
Department of Health Maintenance
  Organization Development
U.S. Public Health Service
Washington, DC

Merrill B. DeLong, Ph.D.
Chief, Educational Development Branch
Division of Associated Health Professions
Bureau of Health Manpower
U.S. Public Health Service
Washington, DC

John M. Dennis, M.D.
Dean, School of Medicine
University of Maryland
Baltimore, MD

Jay Dobkin, M.D.
President
Physician's National Housestaff Association
Washington, DC

Sister Rosemary Donley
Office of Rep. Doug Walgren
U.S. House of Representatives
Washington, DC

Benson Dutton
Office of Research
Health Care Financing Administration
U.S. Public Health Service
Washington, DC

Geraldine L. Ellis
Office of Professional Standards Review Organizations
Health Care Financing Administration
U.S. Public Health Service
Washington, DC

George J. Ersek
Division of Health Services Financing
Bureau of Community Health Services
U.S. Public Health Service
Washington, DC

Marilyn C. Farray
Program Officer
Robert Wood Johnson Foundation
Princeton, NJ

Claudia Galiher
Director, Division of Organizational Development
Bureau of Community Health Services
U.S. Public Health Service
Washington, DC

Stephen Garfinkel
Chief of Fiscal Systems and Analysis Branch
Division of Health Services Financing
Bureau of Community Health Services
U.S. Public Health Service
Washington, DC

Denis Garrison
Research Analyst, Demonstrations and Evaluation
Office of Policy Planning and Research
Health Care Financing Administration
U.S. Public Health Service
Washington, DC

Daniel H. Gashler
Editor, *Commitment*
U.S. Public Health Service
Washington, DC

Mike Gemmell
Executive Director
Schools of Public Health
Washington, DC

Participants

Martin Goldenberg, Ph.D.
Chief, Human Resources Section
Division of Hospitals and Clinics
U.S. Public Health Service
Washington, DC

Matthew Grass
Department of Health Maintenance
    Organization Development
U.S. Public Health Service
Washington, DC

Barbara Green
Staff, Human Resourcey Committee
U.S. Senate
Washington, DC

Ernest Hardaway, D.D.S.
Chief, Policy Coordination Branch
Bureau of Medical Services
U.S. Public Health Service
Washington, DC

Janet Harryman
Director, Division of Hospital Services
Health Standards and Quality Bureau
Health Care Financing Administration
U.S. Public Health Service
Washington, DC

Michael Heningburg
Urban Health Coordinator
National Health Service Corps
Bureau of Community Health Services
U.S. Public Health Service
Washington, DC

Edward J. Hinman, M.D., MPH
Director, Division of Hospitals and Clinics
Bureau of Medical Services
U.S. Public Health Service
Washington, DC

Joan Holloway
Special Assistant to the Director
Division of Hospitals and Clinics
Bureau of Medical Services
U.S. Public Health Service
Washington, DC

Myron Hurwitz
Architect
Division of Facilities Development
Bureau of Health Planning and Resource Development
U.S. Public Health Service
Washington, DC

Kares Jhangiani
Research Analyst, Demonstrations and Evaluation
Office of Policy Planning and Research
Health Care Financing Administration
U.S. Public Health Service
Washington, DC

Spencer Johnson
Staff, Human Resources Committee
U.S. Senate
Washington, DC

Phillip P. Killan
Urban Health Initiative Coordinator
Bureau of Community Health Services
U.S. Public Health Service
Washington, DC

Paul Kosco
Public Health Analyst
Division of Health Maintenance Organizations
U.S. Public Health Service
Washington, DC

Deborah Lamm
Director of Health Programs
United States Conference of Mayors
Washington, DC

Ann Langley
Office of Assistant Secretary for Health
Bureau of Health Manpower
U.S. Public Health Service
Washington, DC

Ann Lawlor
Economist
Division of Manpower Analysis
Bureau of Health Manpower
U.S. Public Health Service
Washington, DC

Richard Lee
Manpower Analysis Branch
Office of Program Development
Bureau of Health Manpower
U.S. Public Health Service
Washington, DC

Bonnie Lefkowitz
Director
Division of Health Resources and Services
Office of the Deputy Assistant Secretary for
  Planning and Evaluation
U.S. Public Health Service
Washington, DC

Jean LeMesurier
Social Science Analyst
Office of Policy Planning and Research
Health Care Financing Administration
U.S. Public Health Service
Washington, DC

Audrey F. Manley
Medical Director, Maternal Child Health
Health Services Administration
U.S. Public Health Service
Washington, DC

Edward Messier
Vice-President
St. Lukes Hospital Cemter
New York, NY

Lawrence R. Mullen
Director, Benefits and Eligibility
Office of the Deputy Assistant
Secretary for Planning and Evaluation
U.S. Public Health Service
Washington, DC

Benjamin S. Neufeld
Public Health Adviser
Division of Agency Development
Bureau of Health Planning and Resources Development
U.S. Public Health Service
Washington, DC

Andrew W. Nichols, M.D.
Robert Wood Johnson Foundation Fellow
Senate Committee on Human Resources
U.S. Senate
Washington, DC

Bonnie Opperman
Program Analyst
Educational Development Branch
Division of Associated Health Professions
Bureau of Health Manpower
U.S. Public Health Service
Washington, DC

Beverly Phillips
County Commissioner
Metropolitan Dade County
Miami, FL

Janet Price
Executive Director
Visiting Nurse Association
Cleveland, OH

Jack T. Reid
Economist, Manpower Analysis Branch
Bureau of Health Manpower
U.S. Public Health Service
Washington, DC

Otto Reid, Ph.D.
Research Analyst, Demonstrations and Evaluation
Office of Policy Planning and Research
Health Care Financing Administration
U.S. Public Health Service
Washington, DC

Leah Resnik
Public Health Adviser
Division of Facilities Development
Bureau of Health Planning and Resources Development
U.S. Public Health Service
Washington, DC

James K. Roberts
Chief, Health Systems Development Branch
Bureau of Community Health Services
U.S. Public Health Service
Washington, DC

Pamela Roddy, Ph.D.
Manpower Supply and Utilization Branch
Division of Medicine
Bureau of Health Manpower
U.S. Public Health Service
Washington, DC

Judith A. Salerno
Program Analyst, National Health Insurance
Office of the Deputy Assistant Secretary for
    Planning and Evaluation
U.S. Public Health Service
Washington, DC

Evelyn Schmidt, M.D.
Lincoln Community Health Center
Durham, NC

Robert L. Schaeffer
Director, Division of Health Services Financing
Bureau of Community Health Services
U.S. Public Health Service
Washington, DC

Leo R. Schwartz
Chief, Emergency Medical Services Branch
National Highway Safety Administration
Department of Transportation
Washington, DC

Gary Shannon, Ph.D.
Researcher, Division of Intramural Research
National Center for Health Services Research
U.S. Public Health Service
Washington, DC

Iris R. Shannon
Associate Professor
Community Health Nursing
Rush University
Chicago, Il

Stanley E. Siegel
Deputy Chief, Manpower Analysis and Resources
Division of Nursing
Bureau of Health Manpower
U.S. Public Health Service
Washington, DC

Morton R. Small
Chief, Financial Management Branch
Bureau of Medical Services
U.S. Public Health Service
Washington, DC

Charles Storrs
Program Branch
Multi-Family Mortgage Insurance Division
U.S. Department of Federal Housing and
Urban Development
Federal Housing Administration
Washington, DC

Ronald F. Swanger, M.D.
Vice-President, Plan Implementation and
  Resource Development
Metropolitan Health Planning Corporation
Cleveland, OH

Alice M. Swift
Chief, Planning and Procedures Section
Student Assistance Branch
Bureau of Health Manpower
U.S. Public Health Service
Washington, DC

Nancy C. Taber
Legislative Counsel
Office of Rep. James J. Florio
U.S. House of Representatives
Washington, DC

George E. Thoma, M.D.
Vice-President/Medical Center
St. Louis University
St. Louis, MO

Mary Lew Tonks
Program Analyst
Division of Hospitals and Clinics
U.S. Public Health Service
Washington, DC

Thomas T. Tourlentes, M.D.
Executive Director
Comprehensive Community Mental Health Center
Rock Island, IL

Plassie Tyler
Program Analyst (Health Planning)
Office of Operations Monitoring
Bureau of Health Planning and Resource Development
U.S. Public Health Service
Washington, DC

Martin Wasserman, M.D., J.D.
Chief Medical Officer
Bureau of Community Health Services
U.S. Public Health Service
Washington, DC

William White
Project Manager, Child Immunization Initiative
Office of Child Health Affairs
U.S. Public Health Service
Washington, DC

W. J. Wilson
Associate Vice-President
Sunny Acres Long-Term Care Facilities
Cleveland, OH

Mary F. Woody, R.N.
Assistant Director of Nursing
Grady Memorial Hospital
Atlanta, GA

Rolando R. Yngente
Financial Analyst
Division of Facilities Development
Bureau of Health Planning and Resources Development
U.S. Public Health Service
Washington, DC

STAFF—AMERICAN HOSPITAL ASSOCIATION

Susanne F. Batko
Conference Coordinator
Assistant Director
Center for Urban Hospitals
Chicago, IL

Susanne R. Sonik
Staff Associate
Division of Health Facilities and Standards
Chicago, IL

Edmund B. Rice
Regional Legislative Representative
Division of Legislation
Washington, DC

Goodrich Stokes Jr.
Assistant Director
Division of Federal Agency Liaison
Washington, DC

Keynote Address

Cost Control versus Public Welfare: The Illinois Experience

Keynote address delivered by Richard H. Newhouse, Illinois state senator

Hippocrates, the father of modern medicine, could not have imagined the problems that beset society and medical care today. The environment is increasingly more polluted. Cities are overpopulated and marked by poverty and urban decay. Resources, both medical and economic, are poorly distributed. The problems facing the deliverers of health care services are overwhelming.

Into this environment has come the computer, with its machine philosophy: Do not fold, staple, or mutilate. By necessity, many hospital employees refer to computer printouts and punch cards so frequently that the human beings these pieces of paper purport to represent lose their identity. The computer card becomes all-important—for admissions, for treatment, for discharge, for posthospital care, and, finally, for billing.

The computer is omnipresent and unavoidable. However, it is also useful, for it permits analysts to study data heretofore unavailable in quantity, quality, and timeliness. For example, the computer can provide data that can be used to develop a profile of the disadvantaged persons in our society.

A PROFILE OF THE DISADVANTAGED

Data show that progress in the United States has benefited ethnic and racial minorities the least. Although these groups comprised only 16.8 percent of the entire population in 1970, they represented 43 percent of the low-income population—three times the proportion of whites. In 1976, racial and ethnic minorities, on the average, suffered almost twice the unemployment rate of whites. The unemployment rate for those below the poverty line was more than three times that of those above the poverty line. The relative gap between the income of racial-minority families and that of white families increased between 1970 and 1974. As a direct result of their poverty, the percent of racial and ethnic minorities who live in crowded conditions is three times that of whites, and the poor are more likely than the nonpoor to live in central cities and nonmetropolitan areas.

How do people in such circumstances perceive their health status? Racial and ethnic minorities are 60 percent more likely than the white majority to judge their health as only fair or poor, and the lowest-income families are five times more likely than the highest-income families to judge their health as only fair or poor. As late as 1960, not only did racial minorities have a shorter life span than whites, but also they spent almost one year in disability. Furthermore, racial minorities had a 40 percent higher mortality rate in 1960, with the lowest-income group showing a mortality rate 60 percent higher than the highest-income group.

Such morbidity and mortality rates are, of course, directly correlated with the use of health care services among the poor and racial minorities. A higher percentage of racial minorities do not see a physician until their illnesses are serious enough for hospitalization. Physicians judge that they treat a higher percentage of racial minorities for severe problems than whites. They also judge that a higher percentage of those below the poverty line are likely to have severe problems, in comparison with those above the poverty line. Relative to need, both racial minorities and those below the poverty line utilize health care services less than the white majority and higher-income groups, respectively. Racial minorities and lower-income groups are two times less likely to have a general checkup than the white majority and higher-income groups.

These statistics reveal that racial minorities and the poor make much less use of health care services than do whites. One reason for this lack of use, and perhaps the most important reason, is the serious maldistribution of health care services in the inner city, where these groups tend to concentrate.

If one function of government is to provide services otherwise unavailable to citizens, then the provision and assurance of adequate health care services in the inner cities should be of primary concern. However, I am outraged at the havoc created in the delivery of health care by bureaucratic bungling that appears to stem from political indifference, if not outright hostility, in government circles. My home state of Illinois is but one example.

SOCIAL SERVICE: A DISMAL RECORD
It would be refreshing and spiritually rewarding to me if I could say that the state of Illinois has a coherent policy of support for the family structure, for its health and welfare. Such is not the case, however, and my experience in talking to other legislators around the country leads me to believe that Illinois is no different from any other state in this respect. A policy of firm family support and concern for family health must necessarily be reflected in the direction taken by the social services delivered by state government, and here the record is dismal.

Social services are the political football of most government administrations, and these services include medical care. The poor, the ailing, and the helpless, lacking an organized political voice or an effective lobby, are at the mercy of those who disburse tax dollars. In these disbursements, mercy does not prevail, nor does justice. A comparison of the dollars spent in Illinois for all the social services, including health care, with the dollars spent for roads and bridges will provide an accurate index of the relative unimportance of human services, which should be strongly supportive of family health and welfare.

The issue of governmental perceptions of the family and family health can be clarified by examining the final paragraph in Section 1-1 of the Illinois Public Aid Code. It reads as follows: "The maintenance and strengthening of the family unit shall be a principal consideration in the administration of this code. All Public Aid policies shall be formulated and administered to achieve this end." That is the law in Illinois. Even those who are only remotely familiar with public aid know that mothers who receive support through Aid to Dependent Children are subject to the infamous "man in the household" provision. If a man is living in the home of a family that has been determined to be impoverished and officially without a male head of household, Aid to Dependent Children regulations require that subsistence distributed by the Department of Public Aid be withdrawn. This is a strange method indeed of strengthening the family unit and its physical, mental, and spiritual health.

This is only one example of the plethora of conflicting federal, state, and local regulations and guidelines that make the job of administering welfare and health care programs more difficult. Regulations from various levels of government must be reconciled so that the job is performed without technical mistakes and so that efficient service delivery is attained with a minimum of paperwork and without the anxiety created by the pressure to serve several masters. It becomes much more simple to fold, staple, and mutilate the human client than to do the same to the unforgiving computer card. Such political manipulation of persons purported to be protected by the state should be a matter of great concern, and I assure you that those manipulated include health care providers as well as welfare clients.

WELFARE CLIENTS, THE EASY SCAPEGOAT
In Illinois, for example, the public welfare budget for years was regularly and deliberately underfunded, requiring a deficiency appropriation each fiscal term to meet welfare needs. This practice had the effect of keeping public welfare constantly in the spotlight and available for myriad political attacks. The deliberate distortion of public aid purposes and the demeaning of its clients became the issue on which many politicians were elected to and retained in office.

This trend continues unabated in Illinois. "Welfare cheaters" has become the new code word for the poor, for minorities in general, and for those temporarily down on their luck. While the use of a code word is seductive to the electorate, what it fails to reveal is the effect of this approach on the nonpoor and their health care. For included in this group are those who are entitled to Medicaid and Medicare, those who have never received a welfare check, and those who are also fed up with welfare cheaters.

Taking advantage of an electorate fed up with burdensome taxation, unscrupulous politicians cater to prejudices by playing a destructive confidence game. They know better. Constituent pressure to contain health care costs has Congress and the Administration in a neck-to-neck race to produce an acceptable national health care plan. Until everyone has a recognized and equal right to health care, the rule that unscrupulous politicians have devised for government-supported health care users will stand: "Heads I win, tails you lose."

The state of Illinois has placed such emphasis on saving money at the expense of the physical well-being of families and individuals that the Department of Public Aid has all but lost its sense of mission. Rather than following the language of the statute, which authorizes "financial aid and social welfare services for persons in need thereof . . . compatible with health and well-being," the department's mission has become that of keeping people off the welfare rolls.

This goal has been reflected throughout the department in the hostile, adversary fashion in which it presently renders service and the resulting deleterious effects of such an attitude on employee morale. Clients are well aware of that hostility and return it in kind. A less-effective atmosphere for maintaining and strengthening the family unit would be hard to imagine.

Eleven years ago, the Illinois state legislature created the Legislative Advisory Committee on Public Aid, which was charged with the responsibility of advising the Department of Public Aid on all matters relating to policy and the administration of public aid. What a marvelous opportunity to reverse the negative trend and strengthen families in this state! However, this is not the road the committee chose to take, and that is most unfortunate.

Instead, the Legislative Advisory Committee on Public Aid chose to become an investigatory and prosecutory body. It has concentrated on a search for fraud and for welfare cheaters. This is certainly a legitimate concern, and some checks should probably even be made on the 300-person investigatory staff employed by the Department of Public Aid for this purpose. There is no question, however, that this approach entails considerable duplication of effort. In Illinois there are presently three separate agencies that seek out welfare cheaters, at an inestimable cost to the taxpayer.

But more important than this costly duplication must be the results produced by the committee in pursuing its chosen mission. In the 1977 fiscal year, the committee recovered some $2 million in monies fraudulently received by providers and recipients. Recipient fraud has been determined to be approximately one-half the amount of vendor fraud. Collections of monies fraudulently received by recipients have amounted to less than $1 million and have led to the realization that some of that "fraud" consisted of errors on the part of the Department of Public Aid, errors recipients could not have been reasonably expected to detect and/or report without devastating effects on their limited incomes. For example, a minor clerical error that benefited a recipient only slightly could result, if reported, in a delay of weeks in the recipient's income, an income that is predicated on the barest minimum for survival.

While the advisory committee was busy looking for welfare cheaters and recovering $2 million at a cost difficult to compute (in view of the total cost of its 11 years of activity), the Department of Public Aid lost more than $25 million in Title XX funds from the federal government, funds allocated for providing the kinds of supports that give families some breathing room and perhaps the planning resources to become whole and self-supporting.

The Legislative Advisory Committee on Public Aid should more properly be engaged in a study of methods to support the health and welfare of the family structure. If the legislature believes, as it insists, on strong and healthy families as the basis of a strong state, then reinforcing families should be paramount in the planning and philosophy of the advisory committee and the Department of Public Aid. The delivery of high-quality health care is an integral part of such reinforcement.

To date there is no evidence that this approach has been considered, nor is it likely to be until there is a shift in the advisory committee's rather curious political history. I say curious because, in its 11-year existence, the advisory committee's chairman has always been a suburban Republican and the committee's offices have been located in a small suburban town just outside Chicago. Needless to say, the welfare problems and the welfare clients are concentrated, not in Chicago's suburbs, but in the city proper and in downstate rural communities. It is not surprising, then, that the advisory committee's actions demonstrate little understanding or sympathy for the problems that exist in inner-city neighborhoods and rural communities.

HEALTH CARE PROVIDERS AND THE PAYMENT SQUEEZE

Those who actually deliver health care services have received only slightly better treatment from the state, although they are certainly in a position to demand better. For example, the abuse of providers came to my attention some seven years ago when I was made aware of the widespread use of factors by health care providers. The factors in these cases were lending money at handsome interest rates to medical and other health care providers awaiting payment from the state for services delivered to Medicaid recipients. Because receivables from the state could not be used as security for loans, medical providers were forced into the hands of nonconventional lenders, whose rates and standards were substantially different from those of banks and other conventional lending institutions. Providers were sheep begging to be shorn.

Many such vendors, physicians and hospitals alike, frequently have their cash flow interrupted by the failure of the state to meet its obligations, thus, for all practical purposes, forcing the vendor to subsidize state services. Strangely enough, it appears that some vendors and some factors apparently received timely payments from the state and others did not, a peculiarity that cried out for the attention of a body such as the Legislative Advisory Committee on Public Aid.

How can the problem of timely payments to vendors be solved? How could payments be brought under control? After six years and much breast-beating, the state now has a computerized program, with a reported turnaround time of 50 days between billing and payment. Curiously enough, that victory for greater efficiency in the system is trumpeted on the one hand, while on the other hand there is a move afoot to take the billing procedure from the Department of Public Aid and place it in private hands, despite the millions of dollars invested in equipment and the staff time devoted to what has been claimed is a cure for the problem.

Similar irrationality has characterized the state's approach to audit procedures. The Department of Public Aid has been known to descend on health care facilities without warning, using gestapo-like tactics to intimidate providers and disrupt their businesses. However, some relief from this policy may be forthcoming. The director of the Department of Public Aid has begun discussions with vendor groups to work out guidelines defining mutual rights and responsibilities in audit procedures. The director is to be applauded for this move. However, it represents but the first step in improving relations between the department and health care providers.

The attitude of the department, a tone set by its legislative policy makers, plays a major role in the quality of service delivery. The adversary philosophy that seems to have permeated the department seriously poisons the atmosphere in which service must be rendered. Certainly monitoring and auditing are necessary, but not as a suspended sword of Damocles. There is no substitute for equity and fairness.

GETTING PUBLIC AID BACK ON THE TRACK

Despite its history, the Legislative Advisory Committee on Public Aid still could be a magnificent vehicle for putting the Department of Public Aid back on the right track. Health care professionals can and should encourage the advisory committee to do just that. The medical professions, with their lobbyists at state capitols, need to support this end and urge institutions to do likewise. Individual practitioners should talk to elected officials, who may turn out to be friends and neighbors with similar concerns about the problems of public aid.

Interest in public aid matters must be shown by people who fit the stereotype of taxpayer. The job is to restore a sense of dignity to a class of people who have been demeaned too long. Look at the statutes. Study the budgets. Appear at committee hearings, especially those of the Appropriations Committee. Put human services on the front burner where they belong. There is a correlation between the health care delivered to families and their capacity to function as human beings.

The Legislative Committee on Public Aid and others involved with the public welfare need desperately to understand the interconnections between the delivery of high-quality health care to the poor, the ailing, and the helpless and the economic health of professionals and vendors. They need also to understand that the delivery of high-quality health care is an integral part of a social service delivery system. There must be a coordination of social service delivery to accomplish two ends: first, to ensure services to all those in need, so that services do not fall through the cracks created by fragmentation and, second, to control costs and eliminate the duplication of services inherent in a fragmented system.

Make no mistake about it. The reputations of health care professionals and health care institutions in this country are inextricably bound up with the fate of the poor and the helpless, for they are traditionally used as a tool to manipulate those administrators, physicians, hospital staff members, and other practitioners of what Hippocrates referred to as "the Art." The quality of the health care to be delivered depends to a very great extent not only on the dedication of these individuals to their patients' care but also on their clear and vocal demand for a change in governmental policy at all levels to permit the delivery of high-quality health care.

Hippocrates is credited with taking the practice of medicine out of the hands of religion and securing that practice to physicians. It may well be time to again follow the lead of the father of modern medicine and recapture health care from the new religionists, those who write the regulations that govern the health care process, those whose false god is an economic philosophy that maintains the appearance of efficiency in the expenditure of tax dollars while expanding the numbers in the bureaucracy and consequently increasing the cost of service. They more nearly fit the description of welfare cheaters. As Hippocrates said, "Where there is the love of man there is also the love of the Art." The "Art" is concerned with people rather than computer cards. And that priority must be reestablished.

Payment for Health Care

The Role of Urban Hospitals in the Nation's Health Economy

Overview presentation by Nora Piore, associate director and professor of health administration-economics, Columbia University Center for Community Health Systems, New York City

Nearly $1 out of every $7 spent for hospital care in the United States is spent in just six cities: New York, Chicago, Los Angeles, Philadelphia, Detroit, and Houston. Spending by the 308 hospitals in these cities accounted for 20 percent of all spending in metropolitan areas and nearly equaled the total expenditures by the 2,912 hospitals in rural and nonmetropolitan America.

These figures underscore the importance of a conference on urban hospitals at a time when a chief aim of public policy is to stem escalating health care expenditures and to find the still-elusive formula that would close the gaps in health insurance coverage without contributing further to the inflationary spiral. These gaps currently contribute heavily to urban hospital deficits and to the fiscal crises of municipal governments and thus compound the mischievous impact of inflation.

In this diversified nation, federal policies must be capable of mandating uniform goals for the country, goals that can be implemented in accordance with the variety of local and regional resources, needs, capacities, and traditions. More than 1,100 of the 5,857 community general hospitals in the United States are located in the 100 largest cities, cities whose populations range from 139,000 to 8 million. Where do the services provided by these 1,100 institutions, the work force employed to man them, the public and private monies expended to pay for them fit into the total health care economy of the nation? Before these questions can be answered, more specific issues need to be addressed:
- Because urban hospitals operate within a complex health care infrastructure that serves regional as well as inner-city needs, how

do their mission, the services they provide, and the resources they consume compare with those of hospitals in rural areas and other metropolitan areas that function in the context of quite different requirements and constraints?
- What is the impact of urban hospitals and the outlays required to support their complex mission on the economy of the cities in which they are located and on the states that contribute a large part of the required revenues?
- What are the opportunites for harnessing the current unprecedented social and political leverage to tighten the regulatory structure of an industry that is increasingly publicly financed but remains largely privately operated? Furthermore, what can be done not only to contain costs but also to accelerate efforts to rationalize the health delivery system, strengthen the health planning apparatus, and increase the capacity to deal with unmet needs by ensuring more prudent and appropriate allocation of resources?
- What role can urban hospitals play in shaping more systematic health care arrangements in the total community health care structure, which is already undergoing profound alterations?

PROGRESS AND PROBLEMS IN THE 1960s and 1970s
While the climate in which this conference assembles is dominated by concern with cost containment, the issues it will consider have deep roots in the events and expectations of the 1960s. As the nation's commitment to extend the benefits of the "affluent society" to the "other" America accelerated during that decade, attention was focused on removing fiscal barriers to medical care and improving access to the benefits of advancing medical knowledge. When discontent flared in cities, both the shortcomings of urban hospitals and the hospital's potential role in an improved health delivery system commanded central attention. Accessibility, equity, continuity of care, quality of care, and jobs—every one of these issues came under scrutiny.

In 1965, a single session of Congress enacted more than a dozen pieces of health care legislation and profoundly and irreversibly changed the parameters for the utilization and financing of medical care. In the next 10 years, sweeping changes took place. While it has been fashionable to lament the shortcomings of Medicare and Medicaid, the data show that, as sociologist David Mechanic recently puts it, "Medicare and Medicaid have gotten a bum rap."[11] Evidence from Ronald Andersen's preliminary report on changes in access to care[2] and the Annual National Survey of the National Center for

Health Statistics, Department of Health, Education, and Welfare, document the substantial improvement in the access of the elderly and the poor to both hospital and physician services.

But in this 10-year period, old problems have persisted and new problems have emerged. Despite increased coverage, more medical schools, more physicians graduating each year, the development of new types of health care professionals, and so forth, the Department of Health, Education, and Welfare estimates that 20 million persons remain outside both public and private health-benefit protection and 45 million persons live in medically underserved areas of the nation, areas characterized by high infant mortality, large numbers of indigent aged and families with incomes below the poverty level, and a shortage of available health care providers.

Meanwhile, health care costs have skyrocketed, and the source of funds has been profoundly altered. From the beginning of the 1960s, when the emphasis was on increasing availability and access to health care services, aggregate health care expenditures in the United States have increased nearly fivefold, rising from $25.9 billion in 1960 to $139.3 billion in 1976, from about 5 percent to nearly 9 percent of the gross national product.[8] The public share of these expenditures rose from 20 to 40 percent of the total.

SHIFTING BASIS FOR PUBLIC POLICY

The search for rational health care arrangements that will provide adequate care at a cost that individuals and the community can afford remains a central concern of American social policy. However, the entire framework for policy discussions of health care issues has shifted abruptly and profoundly. As health care expenditures soar and because tax funds increasingly pay for hospital and physician care, the public's stake in controlling these increasingly visible medical care costs has grown. In sharp contrast to the expansive climate of the 1960s, the current thrust of federal and state policies is aimed at reducing excess and redundancy in the hospital system in order to control escalating health care expenditures and ease the increasingly heavy burden on wage earners, industry, and disgruntled taxpayers.

Other changes have also had a bearing on health care policy. New attention has been focused on the need to care more appropriately for the mounting numbers of those handicapped by chronic disease, mental illness, and the infirmities of old age. Also new in the general picture is a pervasive skepticism about the ability of personal medical care services alone to improve the public health, a skepticism that has been nourished by the new emphasis on the importance of environment, genetic heritage, health behavior, and life-style on the health status of the population.

These trends, in turn, have served, or perhaps ill-served, to compound the general reluctance to allocate more resources to the care of the acutely ill, resources equally needed to pay for education, housing, and other public purposes. It is difficult to say whether the facts have changed or simply the perception of the facts. In any case, these perceptions have subtly altered the character of the debate on medical care policies.

Within this new framework, with its heavy emphasis on cost control, resource allocation, and more efficient production of services, hospitals remain the pivotal target in health planning and health care policy. Hospital costs are the fastest rising component of the health care dollar, and taxes pay the largest share of hospital costs. These hospital costs are heavily concentrated in the nation's older urban centers, where the poor and the indigent elderly are clustered and where the tax base for supporting the competing demands for municipal services has been increasingly eroded by economic decline and by the out-migration of middle-income families.

In addition, the general inflation in medical care costs is exacerbated by the concentration in these cities of the nation's medical schools and medical centers, where the cost of patient care also carries some part of the costs of research to advance the nation's store of medical knowledge and the cost of training its medical manpower. Thus, in many different ways, urban hospitals and the cities that help to support them bear the costs of what is indeed the nation's problem.

A PROFILE OF URBAN HOSPITALS

Surprisingly, data on public and private hospital expenditures by localities are still very scarce, though such information should be forthcoming soon from Medicare and Medicaid data systems. However, by using expenditure data reported by hospitals in the 1977 American Hospital Association Annual Survey of Hospitals, it has been possible to draw the following profile of urban hospital spending in 1976 and to look at this profile against the background of trends in U.S. health and hospital outlays.

The Picture by Numbers

Hospital outlays, which accounted for less than a 33.3 percent of the health care dollar in 1960, make up more than 40 percent of the health care dollar in 1976. Hospital costs have risen faster than physicians' fees, drugs, and all other components of medical care. There has been a sixfold rise in total expenditures for public, private, and voluntary hospitals in the nation: from $8.4 billion in 1960 to $55.7 billion in 1976.

About $13 billion of the $55.7 billion total was spent by Veterans Administration, Public Health Service, and other federal hospitals and by state and voluntary long-term care institutions. Aggregate expenditures by the 5,857 community hospitals that serve the short-term general needs of the civilian population amounted to about $45 billion in 1976. Nearly half of this amount, $21 billion, was spent by more than 1,100 hospitals in the nation's 100 largest cities. Almost 40 percent of the national total was spent by 891 community hospitals in the 50 largest cities.

Most strikingly, more than 16 percent of the total hospital dollar outlays occurred in just six cities: New York, Chicago, Los Angeles, Philadelphia, Detroit, and Houston. The $7 billion spent by hospitals in these six cities amounted to 20 percent of all hospital spending in all metropolitan areas of the nation and was more than the total spent by all hospitals in rural areas of the nation.

Thus, in 1976, the 100 largest cities in the United States, with less than 25 percent of the civilian resident population (49 million), accounted for nearly half of the aggregate expenditures by all community hospitals in the nation: $21 billion out of $45 billion. Almost 40 percent of all hospital outlays occur in the 50 largest cities, which have 20 percent of the resident civilian population of the United States. It is not clear how much this cost reflects the in-migration of nonresident patients, the expensive tertiary character of city medical centers, and the accumulated medical needs of the poor and the aged. Perhaps the historically more extensive public and private insurance coverage that characterizes the city has fostered a less frugal approach on the part of patients and providers.

Twenty percent of all short-term general community hospitals in the country are located in the 100 largest cities. These hospitals account for 36 percent of all hospital beds, 35 percent of all short-term hospital admissions, 38 percent of all inpatient days, and 39 percent of all surgical operations performed in community hospitals. Fifteen percent of the hospitals, 29 percent of the beds, and 30 percent of all inpatient days are concentrated in just 50 cities.

Two-thirds of the more than 200 million clinic visits in the nation are made to the community hospitals in the 100 largest cities. More than half of these visits are to ambulatory clinics in the 50 largest cities.

The 1,100 public, private, and voluntary community hospitals in the 100 largest cities provide training for 75 percent of the nation's 56,000 hospital interns and residents. The 50 largest cities account for 66 percent of total house staff.

Nearly 70 percent of the 28,000 full-time equivalent physicians and dentists, 40 percent of the 473,000 registered nurses, and more than 33 percent of the 211,000 licensed practical nurses who work in the nation's hospitals are employed in the 100 largest cities.

All together, 40 percent of the 2.5 million employees of the nation's 5,857 short-term general hospitals work in these 100 largest cites, and their payrolls account for nearly half of the total $23 billion payroll of community hospitals in the nation. More than 33 percent of the labor force in the nation's hospitals is concentrated in the 50 largest cities.

Other Shades of Urban Difference

Also of interest are the following observations derived from the AHA annual survey data. While they provide few surprises, the precise data underscore important facets of the issues related to urban hospitals:

Urban hospitals are strongly influenced by proximity to medical schools. There is at least one of the nation's 120 medical schools in most of the 100 major cities, and in the largest cities—New York, Boston, Philadelphia, San Francisco, Washington, DC—there are clusters of from 3 to 7 medical schools. The impact of teaching and research on the style and cost of operating these hospitals, on their case mix, and on the geographic origin of the patients they serve is only partially understood. The question of how these costs should be carried in the nation's social bookkeeping has yet to be squarely addressed.

Large cities are characterized by multiple hospital operations. All but 25 of the major cities have 5 or more short-term general hospitals; 29 cities have 10 or more. Except in one city, there are also one or more federal hospitals and state or voluntary long-term care institutions. Rationalizing hospital services in these multi-institutional communities involves difficult trade-offs between institutions and difficult changes in entrenched community habits and patterns of utilization. It also poses difficult questions of physician privileges, competing institutional entrepeneurships, and so forth. Streamlining such multi-institutional groupings poses serious threats to employment in what has been the nation's most spectacularly expanding job opportunity market.

Urban hospitals tend to be larger on the average than hospitals in the country as a whole: 21 percent have 500 beds or more, 25 percent have from 300 to 500 beds. Only 14 percent have fewer than 100 beds.

In contrast, 71 percent of rural hospitals have under 100 beds, and fewer than 2 percent have 300 beds or more. In metropolitan areas outside the 100 largest cities, 89 percent of the hospitals have under 300 beds, and 30 percent have under 100 beds. Both the internal economics of large hospitals and their role within multihospital systems present quite different problems from those that characterize smaller institutions.

In addition to having this higher inpatient utilization capacity, urban hospitals are also called on to fill the gap left by the diminishing number of office-based practitioners in the inner cities. Data from the American Medical Association show that, in the United States as a whole, 25 percent of all patient care physicians are engaged in full-time salaried hospital employment.[5,6]

Comparable data available for selected urban communities indicate quite a different picture in the central cities. They show the following proportion of physicians in full-time, salaried hospital employment: Baltimore, 50 percent; Philadelphia, 49 percent; New York City, 46 percent; St. Louis, 44 percent; Nashville, 40 percent; Denver, 43 percent; New Orleans, 37 percent; Indianapolis, 38 percent.[7]

Available data on patient-origin patterns suggest that large urban hospitals continue to serve as referral institutions for nonresident patients. An annual Blue Cross one-day census of hospital inpatients in New York City, for example, has consistently indicated that about 10 percent of the patients in hospitals on the census day come from outside the city limits.[3]

Thus, many urban hospitals serve as tertiary care centers for a larger geographic area, while they simultaneously provide more routine medical and surgical inpatient procedures for local residents and front-line primary care for ambulatory patients. This imposes multiple roles on inner-city institutions. Ambulances bring the victims of street violence and accidents to their emergency entrances, mothers routinely bring in infants with intestinal and respiratory infections to their pediatric clinics, teachers refer children with learning difficulties, and the indigent aged and infirm come to have chronic conditions monitored and prescriptions refilled. At the same time, patients from all over the area are referred for more complex subspecialty consultations and inpatient medical and surgical care.

Urban America has a higher proportion of voluntary hospitals than the country as a whole and a smaller proportion of proprietary and public hospitals. Fifty percent of the rural hospitals are public-general institutions, whereas only 9.3 percent of the urban hospitals are under public auspices. However, the urban public hospitals are chiefly very large institutions, and the rural public hospitals are primarily very small. There are 1,413 public hospitals in rural areas, and their average size is 70 beds. In comparison, there are 105 public hospitals in the 100 largest cities, and their average size is 633 beds.[1]

Large public hospitals face a special set of problems. They must provide inpatient care for a large part of the population that is without either Medicaid or private insurance coverage. These hospitals also have responsibility for dealing with the intractable problems of drug addiction and alcoholism. Responsibility for the provision of front-line medical and primary care in areas of the city with few private physicians falls heavily on public hospital clinics and emergency rooms. Patients with third-party coverage, and thus the ability to select and pay for private attending physicians, tend to flow to the voluntary institutions where they can be cared for by their own physicians. The public institutions, who care for the unsponsored, those with incomes above Medicaid entitlement but without private coverage, must rely heavily on local tax levies to keep their doors open.

The basic problems in the cities are thus both fiscal and structural. Both the problem and the solutions center around the present and potential role that urban hospitals play in the health care delivery system.

FISCAL CRISIS FOR URBAN HOSPITALS
Despite the rise of federal expenditures for personal health care since 1965, the proportion of state and local revenues that go for health and hospital care has remained practically unchanged.[12] Moreover, the concentration of these local government outlays in the large cities has imposed heavy burdens as health care costs escalate. Because this point has enormous fiscal and political importance, it bears spelling out in some detail.

Public funds now pay 40 percent of the national health care dollar and 55 percent of the hospital dollar. Since 1965, aggregate public spending for health care by all levels of government rose from 5.3 percent to 10.2 percent. The proportion of the federal budget allocated to health care rose from 4 percent to 11.2 percent.[12] Despite the increased participation of the federal government in paying for publicly supported health care services, state and local taxes continue to carry a substantial share of the cost of caring for the poor and the indigent elderly.

While the federal share of the total tax outlay has increased, the *proportion* of state and local revenues that go for health and hospital care remains undiminished. With rising health care prices, the *actual dollar volume* of state and local outlays has skyrocketed. Specifically:

- Prior to 1965, public funds accounted for about 20 percent of total health care spending in the nation. At that time, about 33 percent of all public-sector funds came from federal taxes, and about 66 percent from state and local revenues. Today, public funds account for 40 percent of total health care spending in the nation. Sixty-six percent comes from federal taxes and 33 percent from state and local taxes.[12]
- While their portion of the national outlay fell from 66 percent to 33 percent, state and local spending for health care rose from 7.7 percent of state and local government spending for all purposes in 1965 to 8.6 percent in 1975.[12]
- Despite increased federal participation in the financing of health care services through Medicare and Medicaid, rising health care prices have nearly tripled the dollar volume of state and local spending for health in the nation, from $4.5 billion in 1965 to $14.8 billion in 1976.[12]

These data on state and local expenditures mask wide variations in the impact of runaway health care costs on different types of communities in different parts of the country. The impact of increased utilization and escalating prices on local revenues is, of course, exacerbated in those states where the inverse per-capita income matching formula for federal sharing of Medicaid costs puts them in the 50 percent category. The local burden is further compounded in those states, like New York, that require local tax levies to match the state Medicaid funds.

In New York City, these fiscal characteristics have contributed in a major way to the city's fiscal crisis. The federal share of the cost of health care services administered by the City of New York rose from a negligible 2.5 percent in 1961 to 30 percent in 1975. Despite this dramatic increase in federal aid to city-administered health care services, the amount of municipal revenues, that is, funds from city tax levies, mounted steadily in the past decade. Between 1965 and 1975, municipal dollars for health care rose from 13 percent of total monies appropriated through tax levies for all purposes to 17 percent of revenues raised by the city.[13]

Thus, the impact of rising health care expenditures on wage earners, industry, and public budgets has been especially severe in those urban areas like New York City, where decades of in-migration have resulted in concentrations of low-income populations and where the tax base has been eroded by the out-migration of middle-income families and of industrial, white collar, and managerial job opportunities. The economic recession of the early 1970s accelerated the economic decline of these cities. In addition, with the concentration of medical schools in the large cities, general hospitals have become centers for the provision of the most advanced medical technology for patients from all over the area, while at the same time they have had to assume the role of family medicine provider to replace the vanishing general practitioner.

Hospital costs in these cities have come to reflect the entire spectrum of health care services—from preventive medicine and general practice to the cost of the most esoteric procedures at the frontier of medical knowledge. State and local tax reveues consequently share not only the cost of caring for the low-income and the indigent elderly, but also a part of the cost of medical research. Also, with 66 percent of the nation's 56,000 interns and residents concentrated in just 50 cities, these revenue sources also pay a large share of the cost of educating and training the nation's physician supply.

The urgency of the fiscal crisis in the cities, in conjunction with the number of inner-city families trapped in the corridor between Medicaid eligibility and private health insurance coverage, serves to focus attention on the coupling of two issues: escalating hospital costs and the gaps in health insurance coverage.

IN SEARCH OF RATIONALITY
With the economic depression of 1970, the decline in the base for federal revenues, and the fiscal crisis in the cities, there emerged an abrupt shift in the direction of health care policy. Concern with escalating public and private expenditures has been accompanied by a new skepticism regarding the marginal benefits of increased expenditures for physician and hospital services. Questions are also being raised about the cost-benefit relationships of technological innovations in the diagnosis and treatment of illness that tend to increase resource allocations for curative procedures but fail to produce concomitant improvements in the conventional index of morbidity and mortality.

This trend toward skepticism, interacting with the fiscal pressures that come at the end of an era of unprecedented economic growth, has resulted in an urgent search for ways to contain the expansion in health care expenditures. Hospitals are the most expensive component of the health care dollar. They are everywhere visible and everywhere associated with high technology. They are as frequently the scene of expensive terminal illnesses as of remarkable cures and restorations. They are thus the chief target for efforts to control the disturbing increase in health care costs.

Among these efforts have been federal and state cutbacks in Medicaid benefits and eligibility, soon followed by increases in Medicare copayments. The lifting of the temporary federal price controls that briefly held the line resulted in the search for new control measures in Washington and the state capitols. These have followed several paths: efforts by the federal Professional Standards Review Organization program and various state-monitoring schemes to curb utilization by surveillance of appropriateness of hospital admissions and length of stay and efforts to control the bed supply, first through certificates of need for new construction, more recently through efforts to shrink the system by encouraging mergers and decertification, and most recently through consideration of the establishment of a "capital cap" that would limit funds for replacing obsolescent plants as well as for new construction or equipment.

HALFWAY TO A SOLUTION
Efforts to develop the methods and techniques for bringing this half-private, half-public system under systematic and orderly governance are just beginning. Lewis Thomas, M.D., and Ivan Bennett, M.D., have used the term *halfway technologies* to describe the state of the art in dealing with cancer and other life-threatening diseases.[10] Perhaps that term can also be used to describe the current movement toward a rational governance of the health care delivery system.

In the winter 1978 issue of *Daedalus,* 18 authors were asked this question: "How is the country different today from what it was when Eisenhower was president?[4] The article discussed whether the storms and turmoil of the 1960s fundamentally transformed or only superficially altered society.

For the medical care sector of American society, which in the 1960s experienced more far-reaching government interventions than in all the decades since national health insurance was first proposed in 1912, it is appropriate to ask how fundamental are the changes that have occurred. Paul Starr wrote in *Daedalus* that until very recently medicine in America remained free of government involvement to a degree unheard of in other modern societies. However, as medical costs mount and public confidence dwindles, Mr. Starr sees a gathering determination to "impose on medical services the rationality of bureaucratic organization, of market competition, or of democratic control."[14]

It may be that efforts to cap expenditures and to place ceilings on hospital charges, essential as such moves may be, will be insufficient to address the basic issues of rationalizing the system for allocating resources within the health sector of the economy and improving productivity. By themselves, such controls may serve only to conceal and temporarily contain inflation. It is possible that shrinking the hospital system may only transfer health care costs to other sectors of society, unless more fundamental changes are made to strengthen arrangements for services elsewhere in the social structure. Lacking these, inflationary pressures must eventually both debase the quality of care and break through the crust of controls that are imposed.

Because so much responsibility for all aspects of health and medical care has been given to hospitals, any answers regarding control of health care expenditures must be developed in the context of hospital's role in the health care system of the cities. The time that is bought by cost control tactics must be used constructively to develop more basic strategies.

Two schools of thought exist about the role of hospitals in an evolving and improved health care system. One school sees the role of the hospital in the provision of health care services as greatly diminished. With the shrinking of the system and the shortening of length of stay, the urban hospital is moving rapidly toward becoming a gigantic intensive care unit. All other functions customarily served by the community hospital will be pushed out of the institution, and responsibility for preventive care and for the discharged patient will be lodged elsewhere in the community.

A quite different point of view is expressed by the distinguished hospital historian John Gordon Freymann, M.D.: "America's community hospitals are now coming full circle," he told the Annual Health Conference of the New York Academy of Medicine in 1977, "in the sense that they are returning to the functions hospitals served 1,000 years ago . . . rapidly becoming community centers for the distribution of health care, . . . once again meeting a variety of vital community needs, but they now serve all the people, not just the poor."[7] Although, as Dr. Freymann stated, hospitals are the best building blocks to use in building a community health system, they must be shaped to fit with one another in relation to the overall needs of the society.

The challenge, then, is to bend the evolving framework of incentives and requirements to advance urban hospital participation in the systematic mobilization and deployment of resources and to meet the needs of those presently served and those still underserved within the limits that society can afford to establish for this purpose.

References

1. American Hospital Association. *Hospital Statistics.* 1977 ed. Chicago: AHA, 1977.
2. Andersen, Ronald, and others. *Expenditures for Personal Health Services: National Trends and Variations 1953-1970.* Rockville, MD: Department of Health, Education, and Welfare, Health Resources Administration, National Center for Health Services, Research, and Development, 1973.
3. Associated Hospital Service of New York. *One Day Census of Hospital Patients.* 1961, 1971.
4. *Daedalus, J. Amer. Acad. Arts and Sciences.* 107:v, winter 1978.
5. *Distribution of Physicians, Hospitals, and Hospital Beds in the U.S., 1966.* Chicago: American Medical Association, 1967.
6. *Distribution of Physicians, Hospitals, and Hospital Beds in the U.S., 1967.* Chicago: American Medical Association, 1968.
7. Freymann, John Gordon. Priorities in the organization of medical practice. *Bull. N. Y. Acad. Med.* 54:23-36, Jan. 1978.
8. Gibson, Robert M., and Mueller, Marjorie Smith. National health expenditures, fiscal year 1976. *Soc. Secur. Bull.* 40:3, Apr. 1977.
9. *Health Expenditures in New York City: A Decade of Change.* New York City: Columbia University Center for Community Health Systems, 1977.
10. Thomas, Lewis, and Bennett, Ivan. *Improving Health Care through Research and Development.* Report of the Panel on Health Services Research, the President's Science Advisory Committee. Washington, DC: U.S. Government Printing Office, 1972.
11. Mechanic, David. Colloquim presentation at Columbia University Center for Community Health Systems, New York City, May 1977.
12. Piore, Nora, and others. Financing local health services. In *Health Services: The Local Perspective.* Proceedings of the Academy of Political Economy, vol. 32, 1977.
13. ———. Health care dilemma in New York City. *Milbank Memorial Fund Quart./Health Soc.,* winter 1977.
14. Starr, Paul. Medicine and the waning of professional sovereignty. *Daedalus, J. Amer. Acad. Arts and Sciences.* 107:191, winter 1978.

Tight Money and Expanding Needs: Some Answers to These Urban Problems

Summary of workshops

Almost by definition, a workshop on any given topic is not likely to be a celebration of achievements and good fortune. At the very least, a workshop is most often a gathering of individuals intent on solving a common problem. At its very best, such a gathering can help overcome the inertia inherent in the problem and provide some inkling of feasible solutions. During their two-day course of analyzing the keynote speech and overview statements, exchanging information and experiences, and developing summaries and quietly hopeful recommendations, the workshops of the conference on urban health care delivery touched all the points along the range from least to best.

The problem common to workshop participants was the poverty-stricken cities in which they are trying to maintain a most essential, but currently crippled, human service-health care delivery. In that sense, the scene set in the keynote speech by Richard H. Newhouse, Illinois state senator, and the overview presentation by Nora Piore, associate director and professor of health administration-economics, Columbia University Center for Community Health Systems, New York City, was already familiar to them. The data each speaker provided on the conditions of poverty and the economics of urban health care only served to underscore the seriousness of the problem the conference had been called to discuss: how to squeeze the most and the best from a constantly shrinking urban dollar.

FROM BAD TO WORSE
A short excerpt from the preliminary report of the Commission on Public-General Hospitals launched the workshop discussions in the session on urban resources:

"Local governments in many urban areas today are faced with increasing demands on tax revenues. At the same time, they cannot raise or even maintain these revenues because middle-class and business taxpayers have moved to the suburbs. In addition, taxes are often at the highest rates allowed by law and public tolerance. In these areas, demands for the tax dollar place the hospital in competition for adequate operating funds and capital financing with other government services. At the same time, the problems creating many of these demands—poverty, unemployment, poor housing, hunger, crime, and violence—increase the service demands on the hospital. For example, increased unemployment raises the risks of health problems associated with poverty and cancels employer-sponsored health insurance."[2]

The withering of social services is an inevitable result of the shrinking tax base in cities. Conference participants from New York, possibly the most publicized and beleaguered city of all, were quick to provide examples from their own experience. "If you look at each function in the New York City budget as a proportion of the total available tax revenues and unrestricted state and federal grants over the past 15 years," one New Yorker pointed out, "health care is growing more rapidly than anything else. And yet, it is not, at this stage in history, the highest social priority in the city." Consequently, taxpayers and their representatives are showing increasing resistance to the allocation of larger and larger shares of available local taxes for health care.

Some conference participants suggested that the federal government compounds this problem in two ways. One is the increasing taxing capacity of the federal government, which has "dried up" a large portion of state and local tax sources. The other, and the one more directly related to health care financing, is the differential allocation formula used to compute the federal share of a city's Medicaid expenditures.

Citing Professor Piore's overview remarks in this regard as well as data presented elsewhere, many participants opposed the current arrangement by which "Medicaid piggybacks welfare." As one participant put it, "As long as federal regulations are based on the principle that the federal government will pay a higher percentage for those states that pay lower welfare costs and a lower percentage for those states that pay higher welfare costs, we are stuck with the inevitable result." The result, of course, is that the largest cities, mostly in the Northeast and Midwest with the greatest concentrations of poor to support, therefore have the least capacity for financing health services for those same indigent groups. "Doesn't that suggest that there has to be some change in the allocation formula?" one participant asked.

Capping Costs

Apparently, the idea of changing the allocation formula has not been taken seriously by anyone with the power to initiate change. To date, for example, the proposals for welfare reform offered by the Carter Administration have not mentioned such a change. Instead, the changes that have been implemented have served not to help the cities' poor, but to make things worse. Primary among these changes, as reported by many participants, has been a cap on reimbursements for service. "Rates are now based on average efficiency and average utilization rather than actual cost," said one participant. "The whole theory of Medicaid being a cost-based system is being increasingly undermined at the state and local government levels in order to find some rational way to hold down costs in the face of an inflation rate that is unacceptably high."

The situation in New York City is an example of what happens as a result of this strategy. The cost of an outpatient visit at Bellevue Hospital is $70, which includes all direct and indirect costs. The Medicare reimbursement rate is $48 and is applied to 20 percent of all outpatient visits. Medicaid reimburses $48 of the total cost for each outpatient encounter, and 30 percent of all visits are eligible. Bellevue Hospital is able to collect $12 per visit from self-pay patients, who make up 50 percent of all outpatient volume. In the final computation, this hospital is able to recover only 41 percent of its total cost for providing outpatient care. The same pattern is repeated in every urban hospital, whether it is public or private.

Not only are restraints being placed on reimbursements at the provider end of the relationship, but also fewer and fewer clients are being extended the right of access to care. "Some states are now making it as difficult as possible to become Medicaid eligible by requiring actual copies of birth certificates and many other kinds of documentation that never used to be required, and some of which is nearly impossible to get," one person reported. So the two strategies to hold down costs both impoverish the hospital and cause serious access difficulties for the potential patient.

Shrinking Services

"As the providers who try to serve the urban underserved get financially strapped and pressed, they've got to cut down on something," said one workshop leader. "Obviously they can't cut down on fixed overhead. Obviously they don't want to cut down on their basic ability to meet acute care needs, so the functions that seem to get cut first are outpatient clinics and social services, the whole gamut of activities that we can call adjunct services. And yet, from a rational health care and national health policy point of view, these may well be the most important priorities to maintain."

"The fact is," said one hospital representative from Atlanta, "it is extremely hard to be rational without a dollar in your pocket. A hospital may have a well-developed philosophy that emphasizes preventive care, but it can do nothing without financing." In his hospital, the usual number of outpatient visits per patient has had to be reduced, despite the fact that these visits are currently the only opportunity to prevent serious future illness while caring for a patient's present and usually minor ailment. "It would make little sense," he continued, "to try to put new money into a separate prevention clinic when a full outpatient service could achieve the same objective at less cost and without the risk of further service fragmentation."

Another participant complained that this kind of piecemeal approach has long been apparent throughout the industry, and it has often been fueled by federal funding that causes further disarticulation. For example, Congress has recently begun to consider proposals to spend considerable amounts of money to initiate primary or preventive services. "However, unless reimbursement money, which is the big money, is freed up so that it can respond to the new ways in which these services are provided," he said, "we will continue to have the disarticulation and the program failures that we've experienced in the past."

What starts out being an incentive for practitioners and institutions to improve health care and its delivery ends up being a disincentive. Along the way, providers, whose intentions are good and who are committed to high-quality patient care, "are sometimes forced into semifraudulent actions just to get the dollars to survive." As a consequence, the tension that already exists at various government levels between the desire to respond to need and the imperative to control costs grows worse and pushes the probability of consensus on a rational approach further out of reach.

PROBLEMS OF SHORT-TERM FUNDING

Unfortunately, an overnight clean sweep toward rationality is impossible at this juncture. Even the Commission on Public-General Hospitals, knowing full well that past short-term solutions have been largely responsible for many of the problems inner-city hospitals currently face, has strongly recommended in its final report that the federal government, with some assistance from state and local government, must make immediate short-term commitments to hospitals and programs that serve large numbers of medically indigent patients. The recommendation furthur urges an emphasis on ambulatory and primary care programs for targeted groups of poor.[1]

Though they welcomed the possibility of new government money pursuant to these commission recommendations, many conference participants urged caution. "When programs are developed with federal dollars on a short-term basis and the federal government cuts off support before the local government has a chance to incorporate the programs into its overall design," one person warned, "then you can't avoid the kind of disjuncture that is already one of our biggest problems."

The cautious approach to short-term funding should include several kinds of insurance against fragmentation. One requirement, as the previous speaker implied, would demand that a normal progression of support from federal to state to local governments be built into the new program plan.

A second and equally important requirement is based "on the common assumption that we are still working toward a permanent, long-range solution"; in other words, there must be not only a commitment, but also a feasible plan to build the short-term program into some permanent structure.

If federal grants come in the form of lump sums for specific institutions or particular underserved areas, a third requirement is that regulations must be strict enough to prevent institutions from "frittering the money away by plugging some gap that ought to be plugged in another way." However, these regulations must simultaneously be flexible enough to allow each funded area to use the support in a manner best suited to its particular needs.

Finally, as one participant put it, "You shouldn't use a million dollars to create some new service when the one that I'm operating is already falling apart." Another person suggested that it is, in fact, unlikely that funds would be arbitrarily withdrawn from basic services to be used for some other purpose. "Those programs that were created during the antipoverty years of the 1960s and have since withered away were not well embedded in the stable, ongoing structure," he explained. "In contrast, those funds that were channeled into programs and services that are basic and well rooted in the traditional structure have resisted erosion."

Not everyone present at the discussion agreed with this conclusion or was reassured by it. Some representatives of academic institutions were particularly wary of considering short-term funding. "Each of our universities in St. Louis is currently committed, in the amount of hundreds of thousands of dollars, to supporting programs in the city hospital system that were initiated by federal funds," one said. "Our own consciences and our own images won't permit us to abandon these programs, because they will disappear without our support. As for accepting new programs under similar conditions," he continued, "I can assure you that there aren't very many medical schools that are going to become involved in short-term programs if they know they're going to be stuck holding the bag after federal funds are pulled out."

ILLOGIC IN ALLOCATION
If short-term funding were considered only a temporary blessing, and a problematic one at that, other government solutions were criticized even more harshly by many conference participants. For the most part, those solutions that have been designed to cut costs have become, as one participant from Wisconsin said, "incentives for management of patients to maximize reimbursements." When Medicare reimbursements for outpatient care are cut to 60 percent, for example, a hospital is almost forced to favor inpatient care, which brings a higher reimbursement. "The overall cost implications of this shift are much more severe for a system to tolerate than is the high cost of outpatient care," another suggested.

When an attempt is made to control inpatient utilization as well, through such mechanisms as Professional Standards Review Organizations, then physicians look to long-term care and home care for continued service to their patients. "The result in New York City is a 600-percent increase in home care costs covered by Medicaid in approximately four years," reported one New Yorker, who explained that "more and more doctors are prescribing home care because there are no limitations on home care; it's the only health care service that is not currently being attacked." It is simply another manifestation of the "squeezing-the-amoeba theory," he continued. "If the total cost of all health care services delivered in the city is represented by the amoeba and you squeeze one piece of it, it expands someplace else because you aren't reducing the total volume of service."

The total volume of service and its resulting costs are something planners and regulators seldom take into consideration. The "discovery" of home care as a cost-saving and more appropriate form of care for many long-term patients is only a recent example of such myopia. A study cited by one participant indicates that home care is not necessarily a less expensive alternative "because along with the strictly medical and/or nursing services that home care provides, it adds homemaking services, a form of one-to-one care a patient would not get in an institution." In addition, some patients for whom home care is prescribed are not necessarily so ill that they need nursing care at home; but regulations do not permit payment for housekeeping services unless nursing care is prescribed.

Home care may also be more expensive in terms of total societal cost. If the public budget does not cover all the costs of treating a patient at home, a member of the family may be forced to abandon gainful employment to stay with the patient. Finally, one participant predicted that there is a sleeper in the home care issue. "Those who provide home care services are not yet organized into unions, but this is only a matter of time," he said. If other cost-cutting strategies tend to encourage a very rapid increase in home care utilization, the consequence of the two is bound to be "a geometric increase in cost sometime very soon."

GENERAL RULES FOR RATIONALITY

Having thoroughly examined and cataloged the errors the health care industry has made in the past, the conference participants were at first hard pressed to develop specific criteria for better solutions. They began by generally discussing those characteristics of the traditional structure that should be maintained in organizing a more rational delivery system.

First, "We certainly need dispersed facilities, such as outreach clinics, in communities that prior to World War II were served by private practitioners," said one participant. However, such facilities, whether or not they are hospital-based, should not be developed and maintained entirely at the expense of, or instead of, hospital plants and their services, because communities will continue to have acute care needs.

Second, the best combination of outpatient and inpatient services, facilities, and financing for each community must be left to the judgment of that community. Population and property in cities vary. Each community has different configurations of such barriers to health care as highways, waterways, and population centers. Superimposed on these are the political, social, and cultural mores of each city's population groups. Given this multitude of influencing factors, "no bureaucrat can sit in Washington, draw a plan, ship it out to every city, and expect it to fit," one participant said. Nevertheless, it was generally agreed that emphasis on local planning cannot preclude some kind of guidelines from federal funding sources. Flexible though they should be, standards are necessary so that local planners, federal and other funding sources, private insurers, and others can evaluate a proposal and decide whether it truly represents an improvement.

Third, most of the conference participants thought that the hospital is probably the most likely focus for coordinating all health care services in the community, although many reservations were expressed about the specific drawbacks such a burden would entail. On the positive side, hospitals are already the most visible, trusted, and used health care service in the community: "They are the institutions with the greatest leverage in the health care delivery system because they have the greatest concentration of resources." However, in most cases, these resources are already overextended. To undertake the kind of coordination that is necessary among institutions and agencies that currently have no formal links, a hospital not only would have to maintain its current acute care service, but it would also simultaneously have to become less crisis oriented and undertake the horizontal as well as the vertical approach to patient management. This responsibility would be especially heavy in the inner city, where health problems are often only symptoms of deeper economic and social problems.

As several participants suggested, most hospitals believe that embracing such additional responsibility would be institutional suicide, and, in many cases, they would be right. "Most health care institutions were probably founded to embody the most munificent of human values," one said, "but the longer an institution exists, the more it tends to perpetuate itself. Consequently, these 'caring' institutions will make decisions about expanding services on the basis of their own needs and the feasibility of their own survival."

For this reason, a fourth characteristic of the current structure, financial incentives, should be retained in planning a transition to a new system. "We can get the kinds of services out of the hospital that we want as a nation if we hinge our demands for change on the hospital's need for financial survival."

"There is no doubt that services will invariably follow when new money comes on the scene," agreed another participant. But any kind of money, much less new money, is scarce, and it is therefore not enough to consider incentives. The task becomes more difficult, of course, because "old" money must be reshuffled, some traditional services must be reduced or eliminated, and some long-established and still firmly held practices must be replaced.

The participants agreed that eliminating the undesirable aspects of the system would pose as many complex problems as would maintaining its positive characteristics. Nevertheless, they asserted that an efficient, effective, and permanent restructuring could not be achieved without attending to two negative influences: the inflationary effect of fee-for-service reimbursement and the inefficiency of too many of the wrong kinds of health care facilities. The participants concluded that the answers must lie in prepaid health care benefit packages and in eliminating excess hospital beds or converting them to more appropriate service.

PAYING UP FRONT: PUBLICLY SUPPORTED HMOs
Although prepaid health care services, which are manifested in various forms of the health maintenance organization (HMO), have operated for some time and to good effect in the private sector, only a handful are known to be operating under the auspices of Medicaid. Many conference participants agreed that there should be more, because, at least in theory, the HMO concept should provide what the current financial squeeze demands: cost-cutting possibilities combined with comprehensive service.

One working model of such an HMO is found in Contra Costa County, CA, where a prepayment system has been developed for the Medicaid population in conjunction with the county hospital. "It provides what appears to be high-quality services and at much better than competitive cost," one person reported. This system is competitive to the degree that several unions in the area have expressed serious interest in enrolling their members.

A similar effort in Multnomah County, OR, is operated with Medicaid research and demonstration funds. The Medicaid HMO is actually a broker for its clients, arranging their enrollment in existing prepaid groups in the county or giving them the cost-sharing option of a Blue Cross/Blue Shield Plan. This group also reports improved patient care, accessibility, and successful cost containment.

A current attempt in New York City is somewhat different in that it intends to deal with clients who are not eligible for federal Medicaid support. The plan is to contract with hospitals for a certain number of regularly available beds and with a local HMO-like agent (Health Insurance Plan) for other services and thus cover approximately 100,000 clients.

In each of these examples, the attempt to shape an HMO out of components that do not exactly fit federal Medicaid regulations has been a major stumbling block. One of the regulations that will continue to cause problems in similar HMO efforts is the freedom-of-choice requirement, "a basic issue in structuring the delivery model," one participant said. "If there could be some kind of modification in this regulation, it might help more models to be born around the country and may well be the vehicle that will bring about not only better delivery but also cost containment," he continued. The Contra Costa model, for example, is technically within the limits of the regulation because potential clients are given the opportunity either to retain their Medicaid card and remain in the private sector or to enroll in the HMO on a fully informed basis.

Another problem developing HMOs must overcome is finding the initial capital to establish a prepaid group. In many cases, soliciting capital for facilities should not present an insurmountable difficulty, especially if the HMO is planned in conjunction with the conversion of inpatient facilities to another use. Finding capital for starting up services is another story, however. "When you write a contract with any group," one participant said, "you're obviously committed to providing whatever services that contract covers as of the day it becomes effective, whether you have 20 subscribers or 20,000, so you must have capital to get over the hump between starting services and the first reimbursement income. Many an HMO has simply not been capitalized to the point that it could survive, unless it undertook very strict rationing either of the clients it enrolled or the services it offered." In a sense, such rationing would contradict a major purpose of an HMO, which is the provision of comprehensive care. However, one participant predicted that many cities and states that are already supporting their voluntary and municipal hospital systems through Medicaid should be willing to take the risk of initial capital outlays, "because, from the local government's point of view, you can't be worse off, and you might be better off in the end."

Finding a Better Client Mix

The problems of developing an HMO could be further and significantly decreased if another regulation, that which prohibits any more than 50 percent enrollment of "poor" clients in any one HMO, were modified. However, if this regulation is modified, the other half of the dilemma becomes apparent: the more poor that are enrolled in a prepaid group, the greater the financial risk, at least initially.

"To begin an HMO with a totally indigent population, with the degree of pathology that can be expected from such a group and the degree of unit cost per family, would break our backs unless we had enormous support," one participant said. "Why, then, not comply with the regulation (of no more than 50 percent poor) and expand the group to include a less-expensive population as well?" another asked. Instead of limiting the HMO to a small population of Medicaid patients, that nucleus could be broadened to include a mix that would be economically more advantageous, for example, including all of Cook County, IL, rather than just the city of Chicago. "Studies have shown that, once the immediate health care needs of a poor population are attended to, their utilization of services drops to the level of any other population," this person continued, "so that, if the income mix is more varied, the HMO can absorb the peak demand."

"Even this maneuver would not work in all cities," another person said. In just the one borough of Brooklyn in New York City, for example, there is a population of about one million that could fit the definition of a large area HMO constituency. However, this population group includes from 60 to 80 percent welfare recipients. Because the poor are the largest economic element in this population, and are going to be for a long time, it is impossible to fashion a good income mix. Despite its cost-cutting potential, then, an HMO for such a population group is a predictably expensive proposition.

Less predictable is the cost of somehow providing coverage for the working poor, who are probably the most underserved urban group of all. "Whether the backlog of their unmet health care needs is greater than among other income groups is an unanswered question," one participant pointed out. Some indication of how expensive coverage might be for this group could be extrapolated from some New York City data on a comparable though not equivalent population. "Before eligibility requirements in New York were tightened, the city's Medicaid program was, in effect, carrying a large portion of 'uncovered' poor, most of whom were single, aged, or disabled," one person reported. This group constituted about 9 percent of the program recipients, but because they proved to be mostly an inpatient group, they used about 40 percent of the funds. Of course, this figure reflects the fact that they were being treated under a fee-for-service system and had been receiving care for a relatively brief period.

For Better, Not for Worse

Despite predictions of such high expenditures even under a cost-cutting alternative like HMO, many participants maintained that any such change would be an improvement on the current situation. For one thing, state and local governments are already paying for the health care needs of these groups in some way, either through Medicaid or some other program. Lack of health care at the appropriate time frequently leads to catastrophic illness, disability, or premature death, all of which must be considered societal costs because of such direct payment programs as Social Security and/or survivor benefits.

Equally important, the health care under HMO cannot help but be better. As one participant reasoned, "Even if the costs weren't lower than in the present freedom-of-choice, shop-for-your-own-Medicaid-mill approach, the medical care for the poor and the underserved would improve simply because there would be more continuity of care, there would be some continuing relationship between doctor and patient, and their medical records would all be in one place." Under the current system, the patient typically wanders into an emergency room or outpatient clinic. Because the provider has no idea of the patient's past history, "he has to start from scratch and use every test in the book." Both from a health care and an efficiency point of view, "you can almost not make a mistake in trying to get the poor and the disadvantaged into publicly supported HMOs."

"The only mistake that can be made at this point is to try to get HMOs off the ground without first modifying Medicaid regulations for greater flexibility," another participant emphasized again. "There is talk about grants and incentives and restructuring the system," he said, "yet very little attention is paid to the largest single thing that could be done—and that is to make patient care funds flow in a more responsive way by modifying the Medicaid reimbursement structure. To achieve this," he continued, "we must carefully examine where the inhibitions lie and eliminate them. Perhaps the time for demonstration projects has passed. So many such experiments were so severely restricted in terms of their total number, conditions for operating, and criteria for evaluation that many of them could not succeed and should not be used as examples. What we need to encourage in Congress," he concluded, "is a climate that supports experimentation and permits health care providers to engage in some massive and longer term capitation arrangements with low-income populations, without having to submit to the criteria that work for entrepreneurial HMOs."

HMOs and the Hospital

The mention of Congress elicited comments from some Senate staff members from both parties about the legislature's interest in new ventures, such as publicly supported HMOs, being combined with hospitals. A staff member of the Senate Committee on Human Resources, reporting on that body's discussions of possible federal initiatives in urban health, noted that the committee had been impressed by testimony regarding hospital-based HMOs. "For example," he said, "at Genessee Hospital, Rochester, NY, a true primary care center is operated on capitation reimbursement, with its cost center in the hospital. Data indicate that this HMO operates more cheaply than any freestanding neighborhood health center in the country."

A similar view was expressed by another Senate committee's staff member, who reported the request of one HMO to be exempted from a certificate-of-need (CON) requirement so that it could build its own hospital. "It is not possible for this HMO to achieve maximum savings," she recalled, "if it is not affiliated with a hospital so that it can directly control inpatient expenditures."

TOO MANY HOSPITALS, OR NOT ENOUGH?

The planning of a workable and cost-effective HMO must be closely tied to the provision of inpatient services and the facilities in which they are based. In view of the efforts expended recently to control the nation's hospital bed capacity, it would seem that a new HMO could easily find a suitable hospital affiliate or base. Such is not always the case, especially in the inner city, where the potential HMO client group often depends on only two institutions for inpatient care: the black hospital and the public-general hospital. In the shadow of the current economic crisis in most cities, either one or both of these institutions are threatened with extinction.

Several participants pointed out that the black hospital in any city is often the weakest financially, and the public-general hospital is politically the most vulnerable. The national trend seems to be for either one or both of these types of hospitals to be the first in a community to close, not because the closing is part of some positive plan, but simply because it is one effect of a disorderly drop in financial support.

Former clients of these institutions, most of whom are publicly funded, are consequently forced to seek health care from other sources. Their success is often limited by the unwillingness or lack of financial capacity of local voluntary institutions to serve "public patients," because reimbursement for their care does not cover total costs and, in the case of some ineligible patients, does not cover any cost.

Even if the voluntary hospitals take on the responsibility of these patients, it is just a matter of time before they too will have to find a way to shift the new burden elsewhere. In Hartford, CT, for example, the private institutions assumed the case of public patients when the city hospital closed. One such private hospital has handled the increasing outpatient load by using its endowment funds, but this support is projected to dwindle entirely in a few years.

In most cases, however, some participants reported that private hospitals are not willing to accept more than the 3 percent of uncovered patients that Hill-Burton requires, even though these hospitals are operating at only 50 to 60 percent capacity. It can be argued that the unused beds in these hospitals, rather than those in public institutions, should be eliminated.

It may be true that some of the unplanned closings of inner-city hospitals have been entirely appropriate. Nevertheless, the workshop participants agreed that permitting such a disorderly disappearance of services and facilities cannot be tolerated, especially because many of those facilities could have been converted to some more useful and necessary purpose in the inner city.

A PLAN FOR ORDERLY CLOSING

The city of Detroit, with about 48 hospital closings in the past 15 years and 5 more closings planned, may have the longest and most extensive record of intentional and effective hospital closings in the country. In discussing plans for orderly closing of facilities, a Detroit participant said, "You obviously must first have some good idea of what you want to come out with when you're through and of what it takes to identify the hospitals that are either inadequate or marginal, both from a cost standpoint and from the point of view of quality and accessibility."

Merge and Survive

"The first thrust for us," the Detroit participant continued, "has always been to work toward corporate consolidation or merger, using that as a device both to reduce capacity and to ensure that we have adequate hospital facilities left where we want them." Detroit currently has two such plans in operation. One plan affects four osteopathic hospitals, with a total capacity of 800 beds. Two of the hospitals will be closed immediately, and their services will merge with the other two. During the next five years, this plan will result in a replacement of one hospital with about 300 beds. The other plan involves the city's public-general hospital. The public institution is to be brought into a consortium with large private hospitals. This move would change the public hospital's role to that of a major trauma center. The agreement included the city's commitment to finance the replacement of the old public-general hospital facility.

The process, as the Detroit representative pointed out, is always very complicated, and it takes great attention to major factors as well as small details. The institutions' governing boards and medical staffs must be made aware of all their problems and must be helped to recognize how narrow their options are: either corporate merger or going out of business as a general hospital and finding some alternate use.

Pressure and Support

Often such realization must be encouraged through pressure and support. For example, a hospital that has been targeted for merger or closing because its facility does not meet code requirements may decide to ignore the city's plan and attempt to meet the code requirements independently. In such a case, "you may try to ensure that a certificate-of-need is not granted," the Detroit spokesman said, "and so increase the pressure for the institution's complying within a certain time." On the other hand, if the institution decides to cooperate, the planners can arrange for assistance in code compliance through the state health department. "We do keep the pressure on, but when an institution is ready to go with our plan," he concluded, "we try to provide all the relief we can, especially through the reimbursement system. We assist in handling such problems as capital debt, unemployment compensation insurance, and placement of staff and personnel who are displaced by the change. This combination of pressure and support not only helps us to get to our goal but ensures that we are left with a valuable and strong survivor."

CONVINCING THE COMMUNITY

According to another participant, the success in Detroit has apparently spread the idea of consolidating the health care facilities in the remainder of the state of Michigan. He agreed with his Detroit colleague that "you have to think of every conceivable method of providing an incentive and removing opposition." Often the most effective incentive is the most practical. In an attempt to demonstrate the dollar value of closing marginal hospitals in the state, a study was done of 26 hypothetical institutions that fit that category and that spend a total of $113 billion annually.

According to this study, by closing these hospitals and transferring the cost of caring for their patients to other hospitals, $90 billion could be saved annually. However, the same amount would be needed initially just to achieve the closing, half of it for unemployment compensation and the rest for capital debt, current liabilities, purchase of fixed assets, and so forth. If the front-end investment of a projected year's saving could achieve the closing of marginal hospitals and represent continued savings after that point, he argued that "we should use any financing device available—the Blues, Medicare/Medicaid, special federal funds—to reach that overall result, and I, for one, am not even going to worry about who gets the money."

The need for financing to free a hospital of its debts is certainly a major barrier in convincing community residents that "their" hospital should close its doors. If funds could somehow be found to reimburse that community for the investment it has made over a long period, community resistance might be overcome more easily. "One is almost tempted to encourage the development of some kind of funds, almost like a land bank, to buy back that institution from the community and thus compensate it for years of fund-raising campaigns, capital improvements, and other expenses," one person suggested. How that money is then used by the community, how it is disbursed, is not the essential question; where to find the funds is the problem.

"Clearly, regulations that govern the management of the debt-service problem are not flexible enough to permit innovative approaches," another person pointed out. The solution for obsolete or unnecessary health care institutions must therefore include the modification of existing regulations that are unduly restrictive.

Another solution is being attempted. In Maryland two hospitals applied for approval for construction when only one hospital was needed. After one hospital's request for a certificate-of-need was denied, it managed to win a CON through the appeals mechanism. According to the state's plan, the hospital that was approved first "will add a surcharge onto the patient's charge to buy out the other hospital," said a Maryland participant. The same approach is being considered in another county "where there isn't even a question of any existing facility with a staff to consider; only the planning money has to be paid off before that unnecessary hospital's backers will be out of the business of appealing and reappealing."

The combination of this kind of maneuvering and the facts on which a judgment to close a hospital is based should help to overcome much of the opposition in a community. However, one participant warned that the claim that a hospital closing violates the community's civil rights may be more difficult to manage, especially if it is voiced by minority groups in the inner city. Federal agencies responsible for allocating renovation or rehabilitation funds are often reluctant to deny them to an inner-city hospital, and thus to speed its eventual closing, because it serves a minority group.

However, several persons argued that the question of race must not be permitted to influence such a judgment. If a facility is really necessary to a community and its closing will be a real hardship to its client group, then that facility must be supported with funds for renovation, compliance with life-safety codes, and whatever other needs exist. It would be a mistake to ignore such an institution and "let it die on the vine," said one person, because its slow physical deterioration would be accompanied by constantly more inferior patient care. However, if health care can be provided equally well without maintaining that facility in its current role, the decision to close its doors must be enforced.

EQUAL TREATMENT IN PLANNING
Obviously, such decisions about individual institutions cannot be made in isolation. The combined needs of an entire area of reasonable size must be kept in view as the services of cooperating institutions are planned and restructured. Several participants emphasized that the goal of equal treatment for different patient groups cannot be achieved unless their representative institutions are treated equally. This means that the same cold judgment based on facts must be applied whether closing a suburban hospital or an inner-city hospital. It means that a Health Systems Agency must apply the same criteria to a request from a struggling urban hospital for a high-technology purchase as it would to a similar request from a more affluent suburban institution.

One participant summarized that the goal of improving urban health care delivery is not dependent solely on cooperation among public hospitals. It can only be achieved if all hospitals, regardless of ownership, join their resources. "The only way you're going to achieve a rational set of health care services in densely populated urban areas and under current economic conditions is to get institutions to regard themselves as part of a network in which various levels of care are logically distributed. Any plan that restricts itself to forcing only public hospitals to cooperate," he concluded, "is going to come up short of the mark, which is to ensure equal access to high-quality care to all segments of the urban population."

References
1. Hospital Research and Educational Trust. *The Future of the Public-General Hospital: An Agenda for Transition.* Chicago: HRET, 1978.
2. _____. *An Interim Statement from the Commission on Public-General Hospitals.* Chicago: HRET, 1977, p. 10.

Delivery of Health Care

Accessible and Acceptable: What Urban Health Care Is Not

Overview presentation by Mamie C. Hughes, vice-chairperson, County Legislature of Jackson County, MO

Two facets of health care affect all people, whether they live in urban, suburban, or rural communities, in underserved areas or near a provider conglomerate, or in a location that is underbedded or overbedded. These two facets are accessibility and acceptability.

The significance of one is very different from the other, even though the terms are usually used together. Lack of accessibility will be discussed as a barrier to health services for urban residents; however, it is also a major barrier for those who reside in rural areas. For those in rural areas, transportation could be listed as the primary attribute of the difficulty. When the question of acceptability is considered, it is assumed that cases of dissatisfaction with or the lack of acceptance of some kind of health care can be documented among all income, social, and cultural groups. However, in this conference, the focus will be on urban underserved areas.

BARRIERS TO ACCESSIBILITY

For the urban working class, a significant factor in the accessibility of health care is the ownership of or access to a private motor vehicle or the availability of convenient public transportation. In inner-city areas, a number of such private vehicles are secondhand and thus are frequently out of service. Among the passengers who depend on these vehicles for transportation are those who have no car of their own or who leave the family's one car at home for another's use. The low-in-

---

For assistance in preparing her conference presentation for publication, Ms. Hughes wishes to thank Dorothy H. Johnson, the Greater Kansas City Mental Health Foundation, Kansas City, MO, and former director of the Health and Welfare Department of Jackson County, MO.

come and middle-income workers in inner-city areas often have working spouses. Where there is a second car, it usually transports the second person to work and drops off and picks up children at schools, day-care centers, and baby-sitters' homes. When there is illness, this whole system breaks down until a substitute driver, vehicle, or temporary sitter is located.

Not incidentally, the breakdown of the transportation system also contributes to tardiness and broken appointments. So when physician and clinic office hours are over and medical care is needed, persons in these circumstances turn to emergency departments of hospitals.

Among others who suffer from barriers to health care in the urban environment are the wives and mothers who can adequately manage their households and rear their children while their husbands work; they form the smallest proportion of the population in inner-city areas. These capable women call health care providers for appointments, arrange for transportation, and arrive at the expected hour. Frequently their accessibility to health care is then affected by long waits in the appropriately named waiting room.

Finally, those who may have the least access are those inner-city dwellers who might be described as members of the "welfare" class. Because of the misuse and abuse of this word, I prefer the label "dependent" class. Among these are infants, preschool-age children and the parent or guardian who cares for them; older men and women living alone and supported by inadequate pensions or federal supplemental security income; the disabled; older persons with mobility problems; the unemployable; and the unemployed.

OVERCOMING BARRIERS
Government-aided programs initiated in the 1960s brought antipoverty, Model Cities, VISTA (Volunteers in Service to America), and other programs to these inner-city dwellers. And with these programs came various transportation services, outreach workers, satellite centers, neighborhood health centers, free clinics, storefront service centers, and the like. To one degree or another, accessibility increased by virtue of these programs' two major contributions.

One was the inclusion of transportation services by the health care provider, along with follow-up or outreach services by community nurses or trained paraprofessionals from the constituent communities. These persons could visit patients' homes and see what conditions affected their following the doctor's instructions. The combination of consumer education and transportation assisted in reducing broken appointments.

The other major contribution was the addition of client group representatives to the governing boards of provider institutions and/or the formation of patient advocate groups with volunteer or paid staffs. Although many issues about client representation can be debated, there can be no doubt that such representation helps providers "walk in the client's shoes" and arrange to deliver care accordingly. Communication barriers that had not previously been recognized have been overcome, and in many cases consumers' suggestions have been willingly accepted because they helped raise the efficiency of an institution's operations. Consumers are not competitors with experts in the organization and delivery of health care; they have their own areas of expertise, especially in their firsthand knowledge of a delivered product that does not hit its mark.

LOSING GROUND
Unfortunately, such benefits of increased accessibility are being either eroded or totally withdrawn. Earlier, under blanket appropriations through the Office of Economic Opportunity or the Public Health Service, budgeting was done by estimating service needs. Now, with third-party reimbursements on the basis of unit cost, some of the extras gained through the programs of the 1960s that made services more accessible price themselves out of the reimbursement market and right into the deficit financing bucket. But the current economic squeeze is affecting much more than the extras; even basic services are becoming inaccessible—again.

For example, when community mental health centers were first established, they were intended to serve *all*, regardless of ability to pay. Now, as the percentage of federal money decreases from 90 percent in poverty areas and from 75 percent in other areas, there are problems for those who cannot pay if the center cannot make up the local matching fee income, and mental health services are not as accessible as they were.

So accessibility depends on more than just transportation; it demands that the patient have the proper financial ticket for admission to the needed service. To have the ticket means to have ready cash or a third-party card that is acceptable to the provider. In Missouri, many outpatient providers and some hospitals do not accept patients who are Title 19 beneficiaries because the reimbursement does not cover their costs. As a result, public-hospital outpatient services and neighborhood health centers run deficits on services to patients whose needs are supposedly supplied by that publicly financed pocketbook known as Medicaid. The refusal of some private providers to make their services accessible adds to the vicious cycle. It causes the poor cardholder to be angry with the well-to-do provider and to want government to put a stop to this mistreatment. The provider, in turn, wants the government to leave the great American medical system alone. So goes the controversy of government control versus government aid.

Another necessary ticket for accessibility is an ability to know something about the human body, to recognize and be able to describe symptoms, and know how to find the appropriate provider. The population of the inner cities, especially the elderly, often lacks the sophistication about how the human body works that is seen among better-educated, younger suburban residents. This barrier to their seeking health care is one that can be eliminated only through communitywide health education programs.

Increased accessibility also depends on the health care system's, or nonsystem's, philosophical view. Planning for accessibility demands that personnel be selected and trained in accordance with the philosophy that interpersonal relations between providers and users is as basic as the technology and the art of medicine. This philosophy is a basic premise of the new breed of primary care practitioners. The telephone-answering service, the receptionist, the nurse, the lab technician—all can make the pathway either smooth or full of obstacles as the client winds through the maze on the way to the ultimate provider. Elderly patients must be seen by those who can wait for the slowness of movement, of thought, and of memory as they ask questions and fill out new-fangled forms for old-fashioned people.

An overriding principle that cannot be overlooked is that persons must know who and where the care givers are. People cannot gain access to any health service if they do not know it exists. No system will work well until users are educated about what it can do and what they should know and do for themselves. It matters not if the clinic is public or private. If the intent of the system and its daily operation are functional, the client reaches the target. If not, a horror story ensues.

Here is just one example: A single male worker suffered from continuing respiratory difficulties. He went to his usual physician, who referred him to a specialist and then to a radiologist. He waited for the report on the X rays, but no call came when he thought it was promised. The next day he called his physician when his symptoms seemed to get worse. However, it was his physician's day off, and so the answering service eventually located a substitute physician. The patient asked what to do about severe coughing, which was producing a great deal of misery. The physician did not feel he should prescribe without knowing the radiologist's finding. Later the patient heard, between his choking coughs, that the radiologist's office was not releasing its report because the substitute physician was not the referring physician. The regular physician was not in his office the following day. Apparently, he was not just taking his usual day off but had left the city, probably to attend a seminar to gain continuing education credit hours.

The system surely was not functioning adequately. For this patient accessibility, with all of its ramifications, had not been given a high priority and continual monitoring by the provider staff and the administration of the facility. If this man had not been a paying patient and instead made those phone calls to the hospital's outpatient clinic, he might have been given even less information. Surely, this leads to the unavoidable conclusion that accessibility leads to acceptability. Yet it is not the same.

GETTING INTO THE SYSTEM AND LIKING IT

Once patients are in the system, other elements of health care make for acceptance or lack of it. It is essential that the provider knows how much the patient knows. The staff's ability to choose the appropriate communication system for each patient is key to having both understand each other. If the level of health education embodies some old wive's tales, this must also be taken into account. If a patient hesitates to discuss personal matters with a provider of the opposite sex or if he or she feels the generation or class gap is too great, then it would be ideal if a more appropriate person could talk with that patient.

Many of those who help underserved residents gain access to health care that takes into account their social and cultural needs as well as their medical needs are home care nurses, social workers, outreach workers, and others. Although the general hospital is a major community service agency, its primary focus is and must be medical. However, other agencies and service systems affect individual health and the ability of any institution to meet its objectives. Those professionals in the health care system, primarily the social workers, whose field is to know community resources and how they can be used beneficially by individuals can form a useful liaison for the general hospital.

The hospital should not have to furnish everything and do everything for the patient; it should perform only those services for which it has special knowledge and skill. Hospital social workers can form links to other services in the community. Only when it makes financial and programmatic sense should the hospital have to provide nonmedical services. However, when such services are not available or when community systems are inflexible and unwilling to join in a continuum of care for clients, the hospital may have to find ways to provide what is needed. That is why no single social service plan fits every city.

The addition of outreach workers and similar personnel to the health care team, though costly, increase acceptability, and therein lies a dilemma. For care to be totally acceptable, it must be affordable to the patient and to the taxpayer.

SOME CONCLUSIONS
To achieve both accessibility and acceptability, then, consideration must be given to a variety of factors: to personal and family health education, so that people can recognize illness and injury; to information about care-giving facilities, their locations, and how to use them; to transportation systems; to follow-up; to trust and coordination among providers; and certainly to financing.

This last factor, of course, becomes a bigger issue as there is less money to spend. Lawmakers, health care providers, and the public must find the proper mesh between open access and the financing of what can be agreed upon by all as acceptable. Even more important, however, is the willingness of hospital boards and administrative staffs to make changes that render their services more acceptable, and thus more successful.

Spending money is by no means the single solution to problems of accessibility and acceptability. Rearrangement of personnel so that patients are interviewed by persons who understand them, keeping patients' records in family groups and viewing the patient as a unit within the family constellation, arranging appointments to reduce the number of visits for diagnostic tests, transferring patient information from one provider to another instead of each starting over again, trust between professionals—none of these would have a tremendous impact on cost. They are factors that must be considered if an imaginative approach to the problem is to be found.

The common thread that distinguishes problem solving from building barriers to care is an attitude. The ideas of all who have a stake in the system must be taken into account. Everyone in the provider hospital and the consumers it serves must relate to one another with no less than a cooperative spirit.

Patient and Consumer Participation: Is It Always for the Better?

Summary of workshops

Of all the related issues that workshop participants discussed, the concern described by Mamie Hughes, vice-chairperson, County Legislature of Jackson County, Kansas City, MO, for the acceptability of health care services was clearly the most consumer oriented.

Participants' remarks indicated that acceptability cannot be achieved without a significant degree of consumer control over service delivery. Despite support for the concept of consumer control by many health care providers and despite its imposition in various degrees through governmental regulations, not everyone welcomes its implementation with open arms and without a trace of doubt. Even among those who voiced the greatest support for the idea during conference discussions, two related questions were accorded serious attention:
1. Can consumers, by their participation in the planning process, actually help improve delivery of health care and therefore its acceptability?
2. Is consumer participation, and specifically its ultimate manifestation, consumer control, automatically synonymous with the public good?

NOT NECESSARILY FOR THE BEST
Given the experiences reported by several participants, the answer to both questions, at least for the time being, must be a reserved yes with the emphasis on the reservation. Apparently, several often contradictory factors motivate an individual consumer's perception of how health care services should be used and, therefore, how accessible they should be in the first place.

"Something like one out of every six people in the United States uses hospital services during the course of a year," one participant explained. "However, it's the five people who don't use the services who are really applying the political pressure for cost containment and who thus try to determine what services the sixth person should get. In contrast, the only standard that the sixth person is using is that he wants the best. Given a little time, the sixth person gets well and joins the other five, while one of the five becomes ill and needs hospital care. At that point, the yardstick by which each measures what care should be available and how much it is worth changes. Unfortunately for sick people in this country," he concluded, "they're outnumbered five to one."

"When you're dealing with that kind of phenomenon," another agreed, "it is extraordinarily difficult to apply general industrial and economic principles. That's one of the very serious dilemmas that arises in translating what is essentially a notion of goods to a highly individualistic and variable perception on a 24-hour basis and for the same individual."

It might be expected that participation on a local planning body would foster in the individual consumer an even stronger desire to act like one of the "five against one," that is, to face such difficult decisions as the closing of a local hospital without undue bias. Curiously enough, one participant said, "When it comes to consumer participation, more often than not, he views himself as the sixth person, the one who wants the best." When it comes to cutting back services and costs, his stance is, "Don't do it to me; do it to him over there." Furthermore, this ability to exert formal, government-sanctioned power to get more of the kinds of services he feels his community should have is in no way dampened "by the growing awareness that in fact these are his dollars."

It is this phenomenon that belies the attractiveness and the apparent logic of emphasizing local planning power. "I've heard it argued," said one participant, "that one of the basic fallacies in Public Law 93-641 is that you entrust consumers at the local level with a fair amount of influence in the decision-making process even though you know that at the local level all they can ever want is more. Then you superimpose on the attitude a decision-making approach at the state and federal level that says, 'All you can have is less.' How do we resolve that kind of conflict and still respond to the demand to give the consumers what they want?"

The difficulty is not made any easier by provider representatives on planning boards, whose perception of what they need is no less prejudiced by self-interest than is that of the consumers. This similarity in approach between consumer and provider is probably a major reason why many Health Systems Agencies (HSAs) will appear to "work well," that is, to operate relatively free of internal conflict, as one participant speculated. "If you ask the consumers what they want, they say they want more; if you ask the providers what they want, they say they want more. There's nothing to argue about," he continued, "so everything is handled very expeditiously."

In many cases, additional political pressure is often applied by local politicians. In New York, for example, where some groups of providers have been able to overcome their local self-interest and have been urging the elimination of certain unnecessary hospital beds for more than two years, the invariable response from the HSA members associated with that hospital is, "No, that's not what we meant by shrinkage of the system." One New Yorker reported that the first ones to come to the aid of this hospital "are the state legislatures and the assemblymen who represent that hospital district, no matter what kind of medical or physical qualifications that hospital has."

Who Speaks for the Poor?

Such pockets of narrow self-interest, multiplied by the number of planning areas in a state, cannot help but wreak havoc with state and federal plans for cost containment. At the very least, local planning groups must be told to revise their extravagant demands to more realistically comply with a tight money situation. And so the planning process is prolonged and very possibly the installation of some necessary facility or equipment delayed.

This is certainly a serious blot on the reputation of health planning technology, but it cannot be considered as serious as the continued disenfranchisement of the poor in the planning process. "To begin with," said one participant, "we cannot assume that every consumer on a planning board will be either aware of or committed to serving the needs of the medically indigent. It is unlikely that the geographic boundaries of those HSAs that include large urban areas will permit representation for the poor population to match that of other interest groups in strength."

Another participant added that unequal Medicaid allocations among states will further limit the possibility that state and local planning bodies can address the needs of the poor. "Even basic services might not be included in the state plan under extreme conditions of cost containment," he said, "not to speak of such special inner-city needs as outreach services and transportation." In such conservative areas as the Sunbelt that this speaker represented, "the local government is very resistant in terms of the amount of money they will put out at the county and even the state level," he continued, "so that the only chance you have of doing anything depends on the federal dollars you can get to supplement the limited services the local government is willing to provide for the poor."

To the extent that acceptability of health care services is directly related to control, the medically indigent cannot even express an opinion about how "acceptable" services are. As one participant put it, "They don't have any economic say, they don't have much political say, and on those rare occasions when they are polled, it is under circumstances that don't permit them to really address the issues."

Nor can this group be forced to share the blame for past extravagances and constantly increasing health expenditures. "When I hear the words 'expensive public expectations,' I hear a synonym for that part of the public that's now using services. And that's where the costs are," one participant said. "The portion of the population that is not being served has virtually no health care cost attachment at this moment."

Initiating the Consumer

Finally, one more fault that workshop participants found with consumers on planning boards needs to be corrected before planning can proceed as it was intended to. As one participant described it, "The lack of opportunities that most consumer representatives have to become acquainted with the health care system is appalling." Although their intentions may be the best and their interest may be high, their ignorance of the complexity of the system often drags the planning process to a slow crawl.

"If you try to keep the process going at a reasonable pace, which means you ignore some of their very basic questions, then you end up with the possibility that the 'experts' on a planning/advisory board run rings around the consumer members, who have to run awfully fast to keep up with the implications of decisions that move past the board. There are relatively few people," he concluded, "who are knowledgeable about the health care industry who didn't learn the business because they were involved as providers, trustees, physicians, administrators, or the like. At the same time, it's very hard to find adequately informed technical people who are free of a 'provider ombudsman' bias."

NEVER TOO LATE TO LEARN

Such a heavy indictment of the planning mechanism as it is presently constituted did not prevent the conference participants from being somewhat more hopeful about solutions than they had been in earlier discussions. "I think one good thing about the HSA," began one participant, "is that, in theory, it forces specific areas to at least attempt a definition of unmet needs, which should then be coordinated at the state level with the need definitions of other areas." Theoretically, this approach would provide some local control over what needs to come into an area to complement current levels of service without duplicating services. "That is definitely a step in the right direction," he concluded.

As for consumers being uninformed and the medically indigent being unrepresented, there was considerable agreement that two solutions could be applied to these problems with some success: the first is time, and the second is education. The latter could especially increase the possibility that consumer participation in planning and consumer awareness of the appropriate use of services would greatly improve the efficiency and effectiveness of the health care system.

Giving Consumers a Chance

Several persons reminded their more critical colleagues that complaining too much about how poorly consumers behave on planning boards and about how poorly the new planning process operates is akin to the federal government's withdrawing its support before a new program has a chance to get on its feet. "No matter how ignorant consumers may be at first about the intricacies of health care delivery, it is a fault that usually disappears in the light of experience," said one participant. Furthermore, "perhaps the value of consumer participants in any sort of health care program is that they bring something that is often lacking in discussions among health care professionals too absorbed with intricacies and complexities, and that is common sense."

Besides, the professional planners and the providers have had their chance at improving the system, and the results are open to examination. "In some ways, it's too bad," concluded one participant, "that hospital boards of trustees have not behaved more like people working in the public interest more than they have." The picture at this point might have been different.

Joining Common Sense to Expertise

The goal of educating all planning board members in the practice of enlightened self-interest is to teach them how the concept of local control can work within the constraints of cost containment—to teach them a more organized system of coordinating the various parts of the spectrum of care; to demonstrate the cost-containment features of multi-institutional arrangements, especially if these happen to bridge the lines between the central city and the suburbs; and generally to convince them that they can have more of the best without excessive spending.

This process of education does not have to transform consumers into experts in health care delivery. "We often mistakenly confuse consumer representation as an expression of popular preferences through the political process with the translation of those preferences into technically feasible options," another person continued. The two have to meet and match one another, but they both do not have to be specifically developed by consumers. The consumers can make known their views on broad public issues, such as being for or against national health insurance, by the way they vote. However, it makes sense, in terms of a societal division of labor, for the public to "buy" the technical knowledge that will translate the broad issues into several specific possibilities. At this point, the consumers can vote again, possibly through the mechanism of their representatives on the HSA.

THE HSA: TO KNOW IT IS TO USE IT

Such a logical progression toward effective participation in the planning process presumes a knowledge, first, of the existence of the process and, second, of how to get its attention. "The process of planning and the multiple agencies involved always appear to loom large, like a mountain, to the initiated, but for many inner-city inhabitants the route to it is incredibly complex," one participant said. "To get to the mountain, you have to know where it is, and it's incomprehensible that it could be in 50 different places all around the city."

Another participant compared the problem to inner-city inhabitants' inability to gain access to appropriate health care. "We had a massive, low-income housing project in St. Louis right across the street from the Jefferson-Cass Maternal and Infant Care Clinic," he recalled. "Despite that, almost every night of the year, pregnant women from the project would appear in some stage of child labor. They had never seen a physician for prenatal care, even though it was available across the street and free. They just hadn't known how to get into the system."

Similarly, "there is a marked lack of articulation between the general community and its HSA, a lack that may be peculiarly emphasized by conditions in the large urban environment," said one Chicagoan. "The lines of communications are not firm, nor are they well understood."

Public Relations for the HSA

"The public does not understand the organization or the delivery of health care," another person added, "so they understand the purpose and the workings of the HSA even less. If we really expect the public to take advantage of the HSA mechanism, we must make an extra effort to help them understand what an HSA is and how they relate to it. It's not the federal government's responsibility either to do that for us or even to fund it." Each HSA should investigate and take advantage of public monies that are available locally, public service time that is donated by the media, and other similar methods. "Informing the community about health care delivery in general, and now about the HSA in particular," said one participant, "is an old responsibility that most of us have been sadly deficient in discharging."

However, several participants reported that the responsibility is slowly being taken up in various degrees by the developing HSAs around the country. The most ambitious example came from the HSA that includes the St. Louis area and encompasses health care functions in Illinois and Missouri. In a massive community education campaign, "the agency made sure that every place you turned there was an advertising poster, on trees and telephone poles, in the newspapers, and on billboards." The posters carry a brief explanation of the HSA. They also asked people for opinions and complaints about the health care received and provided a telephone number to call and a source for more written information.

Information for Access

If a public relations campaign can increase meaningful community input into local HSA decision making, it can certainly have a similarly beneficial effect on the community's knowledge and use of various health care and related social service agencies. Often, mounting a campaign requires no more than the exchange of a small but useful bit of information from provider to consumer. Recalling the relative success of what she called "an almost obsolete model" for informing patients about available services, one physician participating in the workshop demonstrated how consumers and providers must share the responsibility for improving access to appropriate sources of care.

"In the mid-1950s," she said, "before we even began the big thrust in antipoverty programs, there were about 90 well-baby health stations in the five boroughs of New York City. These stations had developed a newborn infant referral system by which a postcard was sent to the mother by the hospital in which the child was delivered, referring her to the well-baby station nearest her home. The postcard informed the mother that an appointment had been made for her child six weeks hence at that station. If the mother did not arrive for that appointment, public health nurses attempted to find the mother and child. However, we found that at least 40 percent of the mothers did take advantage of at least that first visit.

"Although this particular system is no longer functioning," she continued, "this same approach of informing consumers about sources of health care could be used on occasions when consumers are gathered for some other purpose. For example, when mothers of new school entrants gather for some preliminary parent-teacher conferences, they could be asked about their usual sources of medical care and the suggestion could be made that they might try using one of three perhaps more appropriate and convenient sources. Short of assigning welfare patients or low-income patients to a particular provider," she continued, "we could use this or some similar intermediate device to help direct the flow of patient traffic to appropriate entry points."

ACCESSIBLE AND APPROPRIATE

"A little more education for emergency department staff wouldn't do any harm, either," another participant suggested. Despite the growing acceptance of emergency medicine and its specialist practitioners, "most emergency rooms are still staffed by the low man on the totem pole or a junior resident doing his brief rotation." Such staffing will rarely provide patients with advice or appropriate referrals once their emergency medical needs have been taken care of, if their needs were indeed emergencies to begin with. A well-trained, permanent emergency department staff can do a great deal to redirect patient traffic to more appropriate care.

Doing Good from 9 to 5

However, most participants agreed that education of any of the parties involved in the proper use of hospital services can only go so far. In the inner city, the value of such education is constantly challenged by the economic and social conditions of daily living among the poor. Under these circumstances, the hospital is constantly asked to handle the community's social problems as well as its medical needs: to shelter tenants who have been evicted in the middle of the night; to take in the aged who can no longer function alone or within the family environment but who, at the moment, have no "ticket" into a more appropriate facility; to admit for a weekend those whose medical problems are minor but who cannot find an agency to take care of their real problems after 4 p.m. on Friday afternoon.

The arrival of these "patients" at the hospital's door is a symptom of the community's failure to provide other means of caring for that type of person. When the question of whether anyone in the workshop knew of a city with a 24-hour social service agency anywhere in the United States was raised, one person mentioned that there might be some sort of telephone referral system in Washington, DC, but that he was not certain.

"It appears that the problem of accessibility to appropriate attention can't in this case be laid only at the hospital's door," one person argued. "The hospital, most often the public-general hospital, accepts these people, but the problem arises with all the other service elements that the hospital must deal with afterward in attempting to refer nonmedical problems to the proper agencies for timely attention. Why are these other resources not more responsive?" he asked. "Why should they be able to sit back and not work on weekends and not have any after-hour coverage?"

"It's a cop-out on everyone else's part," someone else continued, "because it's the easiest thing to do—to send a person to the hospital. As a matter of fact," he reported, "the Department of Welfare in the city of Newark, NJ, does exactly that. At 4:30 on Friday afternoon, they send their leftover cases to the medical center. The physicians can't do anything for most of them but admit them for the duration, until the social service system opens up again on Monday morning." Even a social worker employed by the hospital cannot do much if other services to which patients could be referred or transferred are not operating.

The Cost of Charity

Such shuttling about of individuals with several related problems is yet another example of the unresponsiveness of the urban environment and its institutions to the multiple needs of the poor. However, it also is not fair to the one institution that does respond in this case: the hospital. The amount of money the hospital is reimbursed for being forced to provide inappropriate care is negligible and cannot begin to match its costs.

Everyone agreed that what is more important and more damaging to the reputation of the entire system is the distorted picture this portrays of health care costs. The expense of providing what are essentially social services is charged against a community's health care budget, and when the costs skyrocket, the political pressure and the cost squeeze become relentless. Invariably, the solution is applied to the wrong problem. Rather than restructuring a community's social services, the hospital is penalized for overutilization and its reimbursement for basic services is cut back even further.

Halfway Solutions

In a sense, the establishment of community health care centers (CHCs) has proved to be not only a partial but also a costly solution to the problems of inappropriate health service utilization. Most CHCs share one of the drawbacks of the current social service system: rarely do they operate 24 hours a day. This leaves about half of each 24-hour period during which the hospital is still the only source of care, emergency or nonemergency. The net effect, as one participant suggested, is a duplication of services during part of the period and a competition for the same local and federal dollars because of the overlap.

Keeping CHCs open around the clock and providing them with the kind of ancillary support that hospitals must have would be even more costly, and it still would not eliminate the need for 24-hour hospital service. As one participant put it, "The hospital is the institution of last resort. We damn well better be open when everyone else shuts down."

Finally, the CHC is even less satisfactory an answer to the lack of 24-hour social services than is the hospital. "When a person with a nonmedical problem chooses either a CHC or even, a private physician's office as his entry point into the service system, and the decision is made that that person needs a social service rather than a medical service, how can the health care center or the physician provide it for him?" asked one participant. "The costs of outreach, health education, and social service are not reimbursed to these providers, so neither one is going to have the resources to put the necessary social service elements in place for that patient." More often than not the solution is to send him to the hospital.

ANSWERS BEYOND THE SYSTEM

Many workshop participants found the problem of hospitals being used for nonmedical problems the most frustrating issue of all to sort out, primarily because so much of the solution depends on agencies outside the health care system's control. Several insisted that the provision of social services was clearly outside the role of a health care provider and therefore the hospital should not be expected to provide such service. "If the hospital keeps accepting this responsibility," one participant said, "it will be regarded more and more as the right milieu for social service. This will be a disservice to the hospital, it will be costly, and it will not help to encourage a search for alternatives."

Granted this is true, but many others asked what the hospital should do until alternatives are found. "Whether the hospital wants the problem or not," one said, "it cannot on a given day terminate its usual response and say to a person seeking help, 'Sorry, you're a social problem the city hasn't taken care of, so good-bye.'" Whether this is the role of the hospital or not is a moot point. Because it occurs almost daily, the hospital must determine what resources it can employ to solve the problem.

To begin with, because so much of the problem's cause lies elsewhere, there is no choice but to seek solutions outside the boundaries of a community's health care system. All participants agreed on this point. Perhaps hospitals should be more active in lobbying for changes in social service operations and should provide documentation to local and state legislatures regarding the extent and cost of the problem."

A single citywide or areawide agency should be authorized to coordinate service for patients with multiple problems so that several entry points, for example, hospitals, nursing homes, or housing bureaus, would not be left with the burden and cost of maintaining liaison with one another in dealing with the related needs of each patient. Provision of such a coordinating agency should also be a lobbying goal for hospitals seeking relief from inappropriate responsibilities. "Ideally, the agency should have the authority to coordinate not only public sources of service but also private, voluntary sources as well," one participant emphasized.

"Trying to predict the expense of such a coordinating agency," one person suggested, "would require a good analysis to tell whether it's less costly to let the system run on its own. The cost experience of coordinating Office of Economic Opportunity units suggests a high cost per unit visit," he continued, "and this was probably more expensive then letting the social services function disparately—people just don't get the services, and that's where you save money." Nevertheless, considerable expense would be incurred somewhere along the line, especially when minor social problems turned into serious emergencies.

Another solution somewhat more in the hospital's control is to attempt to change reimbursement regulations that encourage inappropriate care, an effort somewhat akin to solutions discussed in earlier workshops. "Some of the 'social problem' patients we've discussed could more appropriately be admitted directly to an extended care facility," someone said, "but reimbursement regulations demand those patients first follow a hospital inpatient course." Other individuals may need nothing more than a visiting nurse service, but they, too, must first be hospitalized. "We must convince people how wasteful this practice is," one participant said.

COMMUNITY SELF-HELP

Perhaps the most innovative examples of filling the formal social service system gap were reported by individuals describing community self-help projects. This made a good deal of sense to one participant, who explained that "we have two kinds of social support systems to consider: the formal, institutional one and the informal. If we could collectively find ways to make the informal support system (family, friends, employers, neighbors, and so on) more capable, then some of the problems that now automatically come to the formal system—most often in their late, more serious stages—could be reduced in number. Furthermore, he continued, "the formal support system is so bureaucratic and so rigid that it really can't respond in the same way as the informal elements could to a lot of social problems."

Although inner-city conditions do not readily encourage the growth of such informal systems, they are simultaneously the conditions in which informal systems would be the most useful. One participant described just such a community effort, which was initially launched in response to numerous needs that city services had failed to meet, such as lack of public health nurses, grossly insufficient sanitation, and the like. Out of the community's meetings to solve such obvious problems came the awareness of other, less noticeable concerns. For example, one mother hid her mentally retarded daughter at home out of shame and ignorance about proper sources of care for the child's problem. Community members set up a network of "problem brokers" for their area, with each becoming an "expert" in housing or education or health. "The system worked quite well because the problem brokers communicated very effectively with their neighbors, who were often frightened of the system, and the brokers were able to encourage earlier entry of patients into the health care system before their needs became catastrophic."

Several other participants suggested that, with some interest and effort, similar informal networks using established groups, such as school communities or unions or church groups, as a base could be developed. The point is to get community members, through a combination of formal and informal efforts, to an appropriate source of help as soon as a problem appears. This action should prevent the problem from reaching catastrophic proportions when more costly services are required.

CONTINUITY OF CARE

Such early intervention is an essential component of the concept of continuity of care, which is regarded as the ultimate goal of a network of properly coordinated vertical and horizontal units. According to one participant, the concept consists of four key elements:
1. An integrated, comprehensive health benefits package, one that links the reimbursement mechanism with various elements in the health care process
2. An organized health care delivery system (for example, an HMO) that links all sources of care: primary care providers; hospitals; intermediate, extended, and home care agencies; and so forth
3. The primary care physician, who accepts the responsibility for planning and coordinating all the health care needs of the patient and his family, either by providing the majority of the services directly or by supervising other providers
4. Active patient participation in the treatment process, which requires a patient who is informed and who carries his health records with him to each new provider

Information for Coordination

Everyone agreed that an important link in the coordination of health care delivery elements is the information that is communicated among providers as they treat a single patient. "The sharing of each other's observations in the patient record, the accepting of each other's lab results and X rays are essential to this relationship if we are to avoid expending 20 percent of the gross national product on health care instead of the current level of 10 percent," one person said.

Before this sharing occurs, of course, providers will have to develop new attitudes of acceptance and trust in one anothers' capabilities. "It's crazy when you think that every time a patient comes through a new provider's door, he has to go through a complete history and workup," someone remarked. If the patient were allowed to carry his own record with him, much provider and patient time would be saved, not to speak of cost; and the accuracy of the patient's history would be better ensured, especially as a patient gets older and has more history to forget. This would also be an easy way to improve continuity of treatment for that 20 percent or so of the population that moves every year.

The only major objection that could be anticipated by the workshop participants was the possibility of somehow violating confidentiality if a patient's record were more freely shared by providers, with the patient acting as messenger. As far as anyone could see, however, such a method of exchange should not pose any more legal problems than are already experienced in litigation about patients' access to their own records (in the case of psychiatric records, for example). "If the patient carries the record and gives it to the next provider, privacy is not lost," one person maintained. "Every court in the land has unequivocally decided that the information contained in the record belongs to the patient." Once providers accept that premise—and, admittedly, that may take some time—the only task is to find the most efficient way to provide patients with copies of their records.

One participant suggested an alternative that might be especially useful in the urban setting. "I'm not a big advocate of a lot of fancy technology, but if there is one application of real data-bank recording and retrieval processes that could be very valuable, it is in the record keeping of the urban health care system, with its many providers and facilities. Our current way of collecting information over and over is not only wasteful, it can be dangerous to the patient when accurate information is not communicated in a timely manner." A citywide patient record bank could help to eliminate this danger.

"Should the system go one step further and actually mandate information exchange to protect the patient from possible danger?" someone asked. In some health care organizations, this is already the case. For example, the Watts Health Foundation, an HMO-type system in California, includes in its contract with providers an information retrieval requirement. "If a hospital provides a service and cannot give us the report within a reasonable period as stipulated in the contract, the hospital does not get paid for that individual patient," a Watts Foundation representative reported. However, this arrangement would be more difficult to enforce outside a single system like this prepaid health service organization, which has control of the finances and therefore has the power to impose such a requirement on individual providers.

Personal Responsibility, the Essential Link

"Despite the importance of the patient's record in ensuring continuity of care, the information contained therein cannot be expected to replace the primary physician's personal knowledge of that patient," someone suggested. "The record is usually no more than a written history of the patient's interaction with the health care system," this person continued. "It does not address the influence of the patient's environment and his social history on the way he perceives himself and on the quality of his life. This sort of knowledge presumes a primary care provider who is personally interested in and takes responsibility for coordinating the care of that patient. It is the sort of relationship that was inherent in the old-fashioned general practice and that cannot possibly be designed into a fragmented system in which primary care is provided in the emergency room," he concluded.

It will also be the responsibility of the primary physician and his extenders to make the patient an advocate of the philosophy of continuity of care. This will require impressing upon the patient the importance of his participating in his care through compliance with treatment regimens, through conscientious return for further care and checkups, and generally through some drastic changes toward healthier life-styles. Studies have shown that a provider's emphasis on continuity does influence patient behavior. Other devices that have helped have included decreasing waiting times in physicians' offices, which had a significant positive effect on patient return rates.

However, as one participant noted, the success of such modifications of patient education projects in general cannot help but be limited by the lifelong habits of the current generation of patients. For this reason, the system cannot reach the optimum level of continuity of care until personal health care training initiated through primary and secondary education produces individuals who understand the importance of preventive health care and who live and behave accordingly.

TEACHING THE TEACHERS

Apparently, some changes will also have to be made in the attitudes of the current generation of family practitioners and in the medical training programs that produce them. "The major complaint I hear from house staff who are interested in primary care is that things are still pretty much in the same old grooves," one participant reported. "There's not only no role model, but also no appropriate kind of teaching. You're still learning what's supposed to be primary care in the setting of a subspecialty clinic, where you cannot really experience what comprehensive, rational primary care looks like. And beyond that, once you've completed training, good opportunities for practicing that kind of care are still very difficult to find."

Here, then, was the concluding problem. Having formulated a design for comprehensive health care in which all provider elements are joined and the patient knows about and has access to the proper entry point, how should medical and allied health care training be modified to better prepare "workers"? And can the training system be changed so that not only its products but also its presence represents an improvement of health care in the inner city?

Consumer Power
and Medical Manpower

Managing Manpower Shortages: How To Fill the Gaps

Overview presentation by Haynes Rice, deputy director, Howard University Hospital, Washington, DC

Whenever the issue of health care manpower is raised, someone invariably suggests that the solution to manpower problems is more—more physicians for underserved areas, more attention to the distribution of the physicians already in practice, more financial support for the education and training of all types of health care personnel, and generally more money to provide better financial incentives and thus attract more recruits to health care careers.

There can be no doubt that more of any one of these factors should bring the ultimate goal of achieving high-quality health care for everyone who needs it—the rich and the poor and those particularly vulnerable individuals who are in between—a little closer. Nevertheless, focusing attempts toward solutions on getting more of everything may be a little like treating the symptoms without understanding the cause of the disease.

Basic to most of the manpower problems is not so much limited quantities of resources, but, rather, not managing these resources intelligently. This need for a rational, systematic approach is apparent at all levels of the system, from local to national, from nursing aides to the most esoteric medical specialties, from institutions of training to institutions of service, and across health care professional organizations.

Perhaps the two characteristics that are common to mismanagement at most of these levels are a fragmented approach to solving a complex of interrelated problems and a disregard for the careful forecasting of their consequences. A fairly recent example of mismanagement at the national level is the history of the Health Professions Educational Assistance Act of 1976 (Public Law 94-484). Despite its title and intention of "assistance," this legislation could still have fairly detrimental consequences for urban health care delivery, eleventh-hour attempts to prevent such consequences notwithstanding.

LOSING SERVICES OF FMGs

The general intent of P.L. 94-484 was to reduce the number of foreign medical graduates (FMGs) that a single hospital could employ and so decrease their role in American medicine while simultaneously increasing the numbers and availability of American physicians. Two motives prompted this legislation. By far the more visible of the two, both in legislators' public statements and in the press, was concern about the "lower quality" of medical care provided by some of the FMGs. Indeed, it had been discovered that some FMGs were practicing without a license, and there was a great rush to protect the American public from what appeared to be a widespread rash of incompetent physicians. The other motive, I would suspect, was an economic one, borne out of a concern to provide adequate practice opportunities for American graduates.

Even without examining relevant statistics, it should have been obvious, especially to those with any knowledge of large uran health care institutions, that FMGs have become a necessary service resource for many inner-city hospitals, and especially for public-general hospitals. One study[3] of 300 large urban hospitals that have more than 400 beds clearly emphasized this point. More than half of all their training positions were filled by FMGs. For example, 56 hospitals in New York City had 52 percent of their training positions filled by FMGs, 16 hospitals in Baltimore had 56 percent, 12 hospitals in Cleveland had 75 percent, 16 hospitals in Detroit had 44 percent, 23 hospitals in Chicago had 70 percent, and 13 hospitals in St. Louis had 54 percent. Because a considerably smaller proportion, 23 percent, of all house staff positions surveyed nationwide were filled by FMGs in 1977, it is obvious that their distribution is regional and centered primarily in the urban areas of the Northeast and Midwest. These areas also happen to be points of concentration for the poor and medically underserved groups. The only access to medical care for most of these people is through the very hospitals that depend on FMGs to provide service as an integral part of their education and training.

These points could not have been clear to the legislators drafting a proposal for P.L. 94-484. Nor could the lawmakers have been fully aware of projections that U.S. physicians, even with their ranks swelled by new graduates, group practices, and physician extenders, could not fill the gaps left by a reduction of FMGs or at least could not fill the gap soon enough to avoid a substantial disruption of health services to those most in need.

At the same time, the legislators' "information" about the incompetence of FMGs must have been highly exaggerated. The existence of an estimated 10,000 FMGs who have neither been licensed nor become participants in training programs but who *may* be practicing medicine in some settings cannot be taken as evidence of all FMGs' inability to measure up the standards of American medical practice. Indeed, there is no real evidence that this is the case. Contrary to the belief of those who hailed P.L. 94-484 as a necessary safeguard for the American public, studies have shown no difference at the attending physician level between U.S. medical graduates and FMGs.[3] Actually, a closer relationship has been found between a medical graduate's ability to provide high-quality care and his working in a major affiliated hospital. Further, one study indicated a tendency mentioned earlier for FMGs to be more likely to treat Medicaid and minority patients.

Thus, it can be concluded that the abrupt withdrawal of the services of FMGs would deny competent and necessary medical care to a large portion of the population without ensuring an immediate and acceptable substitute. Can this situation be considered anything but poor management? It was only through the last-minute efforts of a few, including some public-general hospital representatives, that such an immediate cutoff of services was avoided. The "substantial disruption waiver," along with other modifications that followed in P.L. 95-83 (essentially an amendment of P.L. 94-484), gave hospitals that would be particularly affected some breathing room and some time to respond to these legislative restrictions on the composition of their medical staffs.

AN OUNCE OF PREVENTION IN URBAN AREAS

The question to be asked is whether these waivers provide enough relief. It is unlikely, because a reduction in the FMG utilization rate of each hospital will still result in a smaller staff, while patient populations will remain at least at current levels. If the federal government can compensate for the loss of FMGs by utilizing National Health Service Corps physicians, the problem may be alleviated somewhat, although it will be difficult to find substitute physicians in the same distribution of specialists that now practice in the entire FMG pool.

Finally, it cannot be assumed that the great influx of U.S. medical graduates who are expected to enter the market in the 1980s will suddenly find practice in underserved areas more attractive than did their predecessors and so eliminate the current dependence on FMGs in urban areas. It would probably be worse than naive to expect such a love affair to blossom without some incentives, which are currently not to be found in much of urban, and especially inner-city, medical practices. And while the use of the traditional form of reimbursement for physicians' services continues, the most attractive incentive, competitive financial rewards, will be useless in recruiting physicians for underserved areas.

The lack of reasonable compensation opportunities is a major cause of physician maldistribution, not only in general, but also in the particular case of minority physicians. Whether black or white or of some other race, almost every physician responds to the very understandable tendency to practice in a community that will repay him well for services rendered. Race in itself is not enough to attract a minority physician to a poor, minority area. Unless the federal government, either alone or with the cooperation of the private sector, can tilt this reimbursement imbalance to benefit poor, underserved areas by making them more profitable areas to work in, it is unlikely that enough physicians will be attracted there, no matter what or how strong their racial identification.

One current federal plan is to locate new physicians in five target cities with medically underserved areas. The intention is to eventually extend the plan to some 20 other cities. However, it remains to be seen whether this plan will be effective over the long term, if the reimbursement picture remains the same, and how much impact it will have. In terms of managing the entire problem, this seems only a minor change.

Not only does the inner city not offer minority physicians any significant attractions, but the pool of minority physician graduates that might be attracted to these locations is very small. In 1970, 697 black students entered medical school; in 1977, this number rose to 1,085.[1] Roughly 50 percent of these students were matriculated in two black medical schools (Howard University College of Medicine, Washington, DC, and Meharry Medical College, Nashville) in 1970. This proportion was reduced to about 30 percent by 1977, indicating some improvement in the affirmative action efforts of medical schools in general. The effect of the U.S. Supreme Court's Bakke decision on this proportion remains to be seen.

What Flexner wrote in his famous 1910 report on *Medical Education in the United States and Canada*[2] is still true of all minority health care. "The medical care of the Negro race," he wrote, "will never be wholly left to Negro physicians." Although Flexner encouraged better training for prospective physicians, he also saw fit to encourage the closing of five out of the seven black medical schools then in existence, viewing their ability to train physicians as "make-believe." The only two he considered valuable are still training black physicians, but the numbers of graduates from these schools in relation to need is sadly insufficient. Considering how minority medical training has been managed, this should not be a surprise. To paraphrase Flexner, it cannot be expected that minority care will be undertaken solely by minority physicians, because not enough of them have been trained for the task nor has the task been made attractive enough for them to undertake.

UPWARD MOBILITY AND MANPOWER PROBLEMS
Without some success in redistributing physicians and locating more of them in urban underserved areas, the problems of allied health care manpower cannot be approached in any meaningful way. Despite physician extenders, nurse practitioners, and other such professionals, the physician will continue to be the focus of the health care team and the initiator of medical care.

This is not to say that solutions to the physician maldistribution problem should be applied without modification to solving the problem of shortages of allied health care personnel. Perhaps the only recommendation that is transferable is to discourage allied health care practitioners from seeking reimbursement according to the traditional medical model. Fee-for-service as a method of financing health care services is inflationary and would likely put many allied health care professions that demanded such reimbursement beyond the reach of hospitals that serve the poor. Aside from that, I would suggest that the allied health care manpower problems are somewhat more easily solved, again through intelligent management of resources.

The more obvious solution may be taken from what has been done in Alabama. Although its purpose is to provide rural areas with more allied health care professionals, the plan used in Alabama can also be emulated in the cities. The state has recruited students through the junior college system in rural areas, brought them through the university system for their later stages of training, and finally returned them to their own communities to work. Such an arrangement depends on establishing a network of regional education centers, often simply a matter of linking programs and institutions that already exist.

The other solution should be even more obvious because it is so close at hand, but for some reason it has eluded health care planners for far too long. For example, it makes no sense for hospitals to recruit foreign nurses, at great expense, when they have large groups of nursing aides who could be trained to fill more responsible positions.

Also, it is not economically sound management to pay unemployment compensation to an unskilled hospital worker whose employer-institution has been closed when a similar amount of money could train that worker for an allied health care role and make him a taxpayer for the betterment of his community.

Hospitals are too vast an educational resource to suffer from manpower problems. Hospitals with shortages of nurses or other ancillary health care personnel should initiate linkages with regional education systems and so provide interested but unskilled workers with opportunities to train for the vacant jobs, especially for those jobs that are chronically hard to fill. This would be a way for local communities to assess their own manpower needs and try to design custom-made solutions.

Of course, this approach requires time for training the first group of graduates. It also requires money. However, some money is already being spent on training the unemployed for low-skill hospital jobs. The Comprehensive Employment Training Act (CETA) now devotes approximately $14,000 annually per CETA trainee, a sum that could be used to train that person in skills that give him a start in a profession and give the hospital a needed employee. Although it has its benefits, CETA is now limited to placing unemployed "bodies" in institutions and having them trained with no particular career direction. Professional training could turn the inner-city unemployed into taxpayers with marketable skills and might help, at least in some small way, to change the character of the inner city.

Many unemployed persons and those in low-skilled jobs are just waiting for such a chance. Some of them are not waiting very patiently. Once these low-skilled hospital employees reach the limits of their demands for higher pay, more fringe benefits, and such, the unions that represent them will begin to view the gaps in the job opportunity cycle as their next bargaining concern. Hospital unions may be faulted for lowering productivity after their initial years of useful reform in management-employee relations; however, I view union concern for wider job opportunities as a legitimate bargaining issue. The lack of opportunities for upward mobility for hospital workers is evidence that management has been derelict, because hospitals have perhaps the richest environment of any industry in the country for developing such opportunities.

A final result of providing upward mobility through urban hospital employment could be the repayment of a long-overdue debt to the inner-city inhabitants who have served as "medical training material." Public-general hospitals and their inner-city communities have paid a high price for the services they have received as participants in the medical education and training system. All the traditions that surround the "use" of patients in this kind of training environment and the policies of reimbursement for that training have made the inner-city dweller a second-class patient and the large urban hospital an institution for second-class care. The mechanism of upward mobility might help the institution, the worker, and the patient win some badly needed self-respect.

It will take this kind of careful forecasting of complex and long-range consequences to bring the chronic vicious circle of deterioration in the urban health care system to a halt and to restart the wheel in a forward, positive direction. It will take vigilance to forestall such "solutions" as those that will be imposed when many FMGs are locked out of urban hospitals. And it will take inventive, intelligent management to use available resources instead of always seeking the elusive "more."

References
1. Association of American Medical Colleges. Datagram (telephone information services). Washington, DC.
2. Flexner, Abraham. *Medical Education in the United States and Canada.* New York City: Carnegie Foundation for Advancement of Teaching, 1910.
3. Weinstein, Bernard. The foreign medical graduate issue and United States hospitals, in regard to P.L. 94-484. Speech at 74th Congress on Medical Education, Chicago, Jan. 1978.

The Manpower Training Establishment: Target of a Changing Value System

Summary of workshops

Conference participants agreed with Haynes Rice, administrator, Howard University Hospital, Washington, DC, that the possibility of losing the current resource of foreign medical graduates (FMGs) looms large. However, they also agreed that the inner-city health care community will have to deal with several other long-standing manpower problems before it can begin to provide comprehensive, continuing health care to the urban population.

As they had considered the role of other health care institutions and related organizations in designing a rational delivery system, the conference participants now turned their attention to solutions that might be found within the training establishments of the medical and allied health care professions. Like all comprehensive discussions on manpower, this one began with the issue of physician maldistribution—how it affects the delivery of care in the inner city and whether medical schools can and should participate in achieving better distribution in terms of numbers and specialties.

FILLING THE PHYSICIAN GAP

To place physicians where they are needed most, the workshop participants focused on a familiar theme: through some variation of incentives or requirements, bringing a new medical graduate to practice at a site he probably would not have chosen on his own.

One participant suggested that some type of service requirement be imposed on all new medical graduates, thereby restricting the mobility potential of a medical degree "either to a specific site for a short period or over a larger geographic area for a long period."

Another person recommended giving the new graduate a choice of paying for his own training and thus "buying out" of the mobility restriction, accepting financial support and then repaying it at some fair interest rate, or accepting support for training and repaying it by fulfilling some previously agreed-upon service requirement. Permitting this element of choice seemed unfair to some participants. "It tends to perpetuate a two-class system among providers," one person said. "If you're going to address the problem of geographic maldistribution in this country, then distribute all new graduates. Don't tie it to a financial mechanism by which you will have access only to those graduates who can't afford the full cost of their own medical education."

Indentured Servitude

Although treating all medical graduates equally in a nationwide distribution scheme might appear philosophically more acceptable, it may present a legal problem. The dilemma would hinge on the elimination of freedom of choice and could become the basis of a class action suit by graduating medical students, who could claim they were being forced into indentured service. Someone suggested that another basis for a suit in this kind of arrangement would be one party's lack of equal bargaining power. "If, for example, a minority medical student had no money to begin with and his or her only way of getting into medical school was through a government scholarship, the government being in a position to dole out money, then the student would in a sense have no alternative but to accept a service requirement," this person continued. "Because one of the principles of contracts is the equal status of the two bargaining agents, the minority student might win a suit by demonstrating an unequal and unfair contract relationship."

Such class-action litigation against supposed indentured service might be theoretically possible. However, it could be avoided. "I think you can probably get around it if you can demonstrate informed consent," one participant said. "That is, if you ensure in advance that a student entering the agreement is well aware of what he's getting into, that he knows he is actually waiving some of his future rights in return for current support."

As for the argument that imposition of service on physicians is unfair to them as a group if similar requirements are not imposed on other professions, several participants had a ready response. In comparison to lawyers and engineers, physicians "are a very select class of individuals," they said, "a class that can rightly be described as a national resource." The federal government and, to a lesser degree, state governments invest amounts of money in the development and maintenance of this resource "either directly through subsidies of education or indirectly through payments for service." Especially when the investment is made directly through support of an individual's training, the nation has a right to ask for a fair return on that investment.

Quality and the Unwilling Student

Not all objections to enforced physician distribution were so easily answered. One of the more troubling problems to be expected from required services is lower-quality care. "Having served in a number of inner-city hospitals," one person said, "I've seen the implications of people serving time rather than serving people. This situation is almost inevitable when you place large numbers of providers who are not wedded to the idea of serving a certain population in that kind of work setting. If physician redistribution is to provide anything more than minimal-quality health care to the inner city," this person continued, "it must be accompanied by efforts to bring inner-city health care facilities up to a standard that most new practitioners would find acceptable, if not attractive. Otherwise, we're just doing part of the job," he concluded.

In addition to fostering lower-quality care, neglecting the improvement of the underserved health care setting is likely to encourage a repetition of others' experience with physician distribution schemes. "Reports from Puerto Rico, Yugoslavia, and elsewhere," said one participant, "indicate that their new physicians fulfill their service arrangements in the hinterlands but that they have never been accused of practicing good-quality, comprehensive kinds of care in the situation." What is more, when their service is completed, they quickly abandon the service setting and "head for the more attractive environment, where many of them choose to drive cabs, if they can't find medical positions, rather than return to medicine in the hinterlands."

Once a GP, Always a GP?

If there is little evidence to support the concept of restricting geographic mobility, then why not try a more voluntary approach. "If all the specialty training bodies would require new graduates to have a period of general-practice experience before they qualify to enter the specialty training program, they would have the option to go anywhere in the country," someone suggested. This arrangement would not indenture them to a particular branch of service or to a specific location, but it would encourage new practitioners to seek practice sites in a wider variety of settings because the most attractive environments could not possibly support them all. If the choice is made voluntarily, "a good many of these doctors would find it comfortable and interesting to stay in those locations. Having been there for a year or two, they would have developed some roots and some local interests—probably enough to have a significant impact on the maldistribution problem."

"This speculation might be a bit more optimistic than new evidence would indicate," another participant said. Certainly a sizable increase in the number of physicians in the primary care field would alleviate some of the maldistribution. Furthermore, "the figures look very good for entry of recent graduates into family medicine and primary care residencies." However, recently published data suggest that these graduates are not all going to remain generalists in medicine.[1] For example, a large portion take two years of a family medicine residency and then a year of cardiology or three years of general internal medicine and two years of gastrointestinal fellowship. "So maybe the idea of putting a larger number of graduates into general practice may work, but only for a short time," this participant suggested.

NO HEROES IN FAMILY PRACTICE

Why is commitment to treating the "average patient" so short lived, even among those students who enter medical school with the most selfless dedication? Although society in general must bear much of the blame for discouraging the values that lead individuals to work in less-than-affluent surroundings, all the participants agreed that the medical school environment is a major influence in turning potential generalists away from their original intent and toward the newly apparent advantages of the superspecialist. In the real environment of clinical training, a medical school's support of the family practice concept too often becomes mere lip service.

"If we take a group of medical students and preach family practice and primary care to them while the role models they see in their clinical years are specialists who are well regarded by their colleagues, financially well off, and worshipped by their patients," said one medical school administrator, "the students quickly make the comparison, to the detriment of family practice. Even if we try to provide them with good primary care training environments, they must conclude that at this point in the evolution of family practice the difference between the two choices is quite stark."

The difference does not lie only in the kind of future a medical student can anticipate by choosing one route rather than the other. Family practice residents can also expect to be second-class citizens in training. Most family practice curriculums require residents to complete a number of brief rotations through various specialties, for example, pediatrics, where they learn and perform side by side with the residents of that specialty. The latter group has a much longer time to amass the experience that the family practice residents must acquire in a few short months. "It is this difference," he continued, "that is the basis for the second-class citizenship and that prevents the family practice resident from ever being the equal of other specialty residents either in knowledge or skill. It's amazing how much fortitude family practice residents must have in order to undergo such inevitably unpleasant comparisons four to five times a year."

Someone else suggested that the situation may also be a portent of medicolegal problems in the resident's future; for example, how will the family practitioner's level of care stand up under scrutiny if his knowledge and skills are judged by the same criteria that are applied to various specialists?

Building Role Models

Some participants considered the choice of specialty over family practice an almost inevitable result in the natural progression of medical training. "Even if we took all the existing role models out of the way and let it start all over again," one said, "we would see that the tendency of medical school graduates is toward acute care and specialty practice. It's like football training: you don't like to do the calisthenics, but you love the scrimmage, because it's more exciting." Others disagreed, and their choice for a way to encourage change was enhancing the role model.

To begin with, primary care physicians who spend a lot of time in clinical service while also on a medical school faculty "are a sorry lot when it comes to being promoted to a full-time faculty position," one school administrator pointed out. "They simply don't measure up to the normal academic criteria, and the executive faculty committee members usually look down their noses at a suggested promotion. As a solution to the problems we have created a new category of full-time faculty, called 'professor of clinical medicine,' that has different criteria for promotion," he continued, "and we are attracting a lot of good young people." They are respected by their colleagues, they are well paid, and they can hold their own in attracting students to family practice.

An additional fault in current family practice training that can be corrected is the design of curriculum and training essentials. Because family practice is a relatively new area of medical training, its development in medical school departments has depended on family physicians with little experience in academia. Initially, they had little idea of the best way to write training essentials and, consequently, developed the series of short rotations. Besides the drawback that the participants had previously pointed out in discussing this arrangement, one participant emphasized that short rotations do not permit the resident to acquire an increasing level of responsibility. Furthermore, short rotations tend to perpetuate the acute-care perspective and neglect primary care, a traditional fault in all the established medical specialties.

"I see now that the whole basis of my residency training program was the inpatient unit and that ambulatory care was given secondary treatment," a physician participant recalled. "If you structured your curriculum on primary care and gave secondary and tertiary care the attention it deserves in proportion to all patient care needs," he continued, "you should not end up spending four to six months of a three-year pediatric training program in the neonatal intensive care unit. Such an imbalance in training emphasis does not reflect what even a specialist like the pediatrician will be doing in practice," he concluded. As a result, the new practitioner is not prepared to handle the kinds of medical needs that are most prevalent in actual patient care, especially in the inner city.

Several participants maintained that the obligation to reverse this trend in developing appropriate family practice curriculums must lie nowhere else but with the medical schools. "The leadership in medical schools has not given the problem sufficient recognition in the past," and now they must accept the responsibility and take action. However, "if you leave it to the schools," one administrator cautioned, "I'm afraid the only drawing card we have in our hand forces us back into emphasizing specialties again. That's the one thing that we have to attract the good student to an inner-city medical school and the only thing that seems to attract him enough to stay at least through residency. If emphasis is placed instead on ambulatory or primary care, which puts the student now and in the future at the lower end of the economic totem pole," he continued, "the prospects are not attractive enough for that student to put up with the problems of living and raising a family in the inner city."

So the drawing cards that medical schools have used turn out to be the wrong ones for accomplishing a more balanced specialty distribution. Even the occasional success is often very limited. Students who choose family practice residencies in the inner city seldom choose family practice there after completing their training. If they choose to remain in that environment at all, they become medical school faculty members and avoid contact with the community.

Building Practice Models

Left to itself, the situation certainly cannot be expected to improve spontaneously, and medical schools must be more inventive in the solutions they design for the inner city. For example, one medical school administrator reported, "We've developed career appointments that are attached to the medical school but whose primary obligation is to develop a community service program, a nucleus around which other physicians can be attracted. We expect to recruit high-powered professors and to help them build the reputation of these centers as excellent places for ambulatory care. We think young doctors will want to become a part of this kind of program."

Another possibility was suggested by a former practitioner-turned-administrator, who described his personal experience with a mixed-specialty group practice (general internal medicine, pediatrics, and general surgery) as "a very effective way to deliver primary care and a model teaching situation." The group maintains about 12 practitioners, it continues to prosper, "and students stand in line for the chance at the preceptor positions. They like this method tremendously," he reported. Although no one could identify a specific working model, it was further suggested that this mixed-specialty approach might be combined with the principles of a health maintenance organization for yet another realistic model in which students might be trained in family practice.

Even less-structured arrangements may have some success in attracting students to primary care practice in the city, especially if the medical school faculty is committed to such arrangements. "If the medical school and its faculty members share the philosophy of service to the community, then faculty members, no matter what their specialty, will convey their values to the students and will have a broad influence on how students view their responsibilities when they become practitioners," maintained one participant.

For example, another person reported that minority faculty members who also practice in the community around a New Jersey medical school appear to have considerable influence in convincing students, in particular, minority students, to stay in that community after training. In cooperation with a committee of other leading black citizens, they make a point of demonstrating to students who are completing their residencies the advantages of practicing within that social structure.

A similar success can be anticipated from the social medicine program at the Montefiore Hospital and Health Center in the Bronx borough of New York City. As a result of careful recruiting efforts, a hospital representative reported that the current class of residents promises to yield some dozen new practitioners who are committed to serving the South Bronx area, "a community that leaves a lot to be desired in terms of the social amenities of life." The leadership of the hospital has incorporated this kind of service attitude into "their philosophy of running their education programs for the past 25 years," someone else said, "and they've also been careful in selecting the kinds of students who will respond positively to this approach. That's why they get the results."

Lest this example appear too rosy, another person cautioned that the hospital was realistic enough to know that some additional attractions might be useful. It provided a structured program in which the new practitioners could work; moonlighting opportunities in the neighboring affluent community, where most of the residents have established their households; and some other "embellishments." "Doing additional things to make the experience attractive may be a lesson to the rest of us who are looking for answers," this person concluded. "If it works, don't knock it."

Apparently, then, a combined appeal to idealism and to the desire for at least a comfortable livelihood promises to be most effective in attracting practitioners to the inner city, or to any underserved area for that matter. Dependence on the student selection process alone is an unreliable tool for discovering the dedicated few who are most likely to choose urban practice among the poor. Students' interests and intentions seem to change several times and quite drastically during the course of training.

A few studies indicate that establishing a kind of psychological tie between a student and a community is one device that seems to have made at least a small difference. For example, a certain number of admission slots can be allocated to students from particular urban counties, with the unwritten understanding that the students would return there for practice, at least for a time.

On the other hand, flooding the medical schools through open enrollment in hopes of eventually retaining more physicians for the inner city did not win many votes of confidence from workshop participants. Most of the students who would be accepted because of such an admission policy would be incapable of meeting training criteria. Those who succeeded in completing their training would not necessarily be any more committed to inner-city service than would the average graduate.

"The problems of living and practicing in the inner city tend to be equally strong deterrents to choosing that as a work environment, whether you were brought up in that environment or not," someone suggested. Comfortable living conditions, good schools, and a safe, affordable, and stimulating practice setting—all these are difficult to find in the inner city, especially under conditions of falling reimbursements and service shrinkage."

"No matter how much of the responsibility we try to put on the shoulders of medical schools for not doing their share in stimulating efforts toward inner-city primary care practice, we may be asking too much of them," one participant said. "Academic medicine has had as much trouble getting financing for its work as have hospitals," he continued. "People don't mind being good, but they don't want to be good for nothing. They want and need to get paid, and we can't blame anyone for that."

FUNDING MECHANISMS ENDANGERED

As is true of most endeavors in health care delivery, the conference participants concluded that significant changes in the medical training establishment would have to be accompanied, if not preceded, by some bolstering and expansion of current financing mechanisms for education. They noted with some alarm that traditional support, much of it in the form of payment for clinical service rendered in the course of training, is being threatened by those third-party payers and others who claim that the sick should not bear the burden of financing medical and allied health care manpower education. The threat has become a reality to the degree that payments for services have been sharply reduced, especially in publicly funded programs. This, in turn, has depleted the revenues that would normally be used to support house staff in inner-city hospitals.

Besides disabling current service programs, everyone agreed that such real and threatened cutbacks demonstrate an amazing lack of foresight. "Just as every business and industry in the United States sets aside a portion of its expenditures for the development of people and ideas," one person said, "there should similarly be a social decision that a portion of the health insurance premium should be used to pay for the development of skills and knowledge among the people who are going to provide medical and related health care in the future. Everyone should be able to understand society's need for this kind of investment."

"Another convincing argument for retaining the current payment mechanism," someone added, "is that the quality of care in an affiliated or teaching hospital is invariably better because of the close relationship of service and education." This is a benefit that patients can reap now, without waiting for a future payoff.

An Inseparable Combination

Despite the logic of these arguments, many third-party payers will continue to apply pressure to change the current funding mechanism. One alternative that they suggest is the delineation between costs of service and costs of training in an affiliated hospital, a move that several participants considered a dangerous ploy because it could be a first step to singling out costs that would not be reimbursed.

Most of the participants agreed that identifying such costs would be an arbitrary process at best. "The line between service and training is often very thin," one said. "First of all, education and service and research are joint products, and one of the reasons you can't separate one from the other is that they are going on simultaneously in any lively program, whether it's internal medicine or nursing or medical technology. They reinforce one another's quality and momentum." Second, in terms of simple cost accounting, the task of separating training from service costs and arriving at real figures is nearly impossible, and, as some participants had suggested previously, the threat of eliminating reimbursement for the training portion can then become a reality.

One person reported that the state of New York is a ready example. "In 1976, they somehow identified education costs in all of the hospitals with Medicaid and Blue Cross reimbursement, and each year since then have proceeded to automatically disallow 10 percent of the cost that was attributable to education. There's no satisfactory way of responding to that, because next year you'll just have 10 percent more taken from the 90 percent that's left. The intent of the state in this case was to force the hospitals to find some other source of funding," he continued, "and the first source the hospitals tried was the medical schools, but to no avail."

What other alternative might be available to hospitals if this trend continues? Might the federal government be prevailed upon to undertake the education portion if third-party payers are successful in their pressure to separate service from training costs? Depending on the usual vagaries of politics and public pressure, initial funding might be available through some new federal program. However, "the history of federal funding is notoriously insecure," one person reminded the more optimistic workshop participants. "It has been unreliable both in its appropriations and its expenditures on any prolonged basis." Education must be based on a reasonably sustained source of support, not on a "swinging from ditch to ditch as you change administrations or fads in policy," he continued. "Capitation, for example, is going to go out the window, and the same will eventually happen with most other federally funded programs," he predicted, "because the government has none of the responsibility for carrying out training over the long haul or for the appropriateness and competence of the products of that training. Finally, inasmuch as money follows money, lost federal appropriations also tend to dry up other sources of funds," he concluded, "and the combination of the two is not good public policy."

Another participant granted that federal support of almost any activity has these inherent drawbacks. Nevertheless, federal funds, in combination with financial support from other major third-party payers, have been the only large and long-term sources of funds for many training programs. So "it is still necessary to continue to encourage the government to support training, especially in some of the more nontraditional approaches to health care delivery, such as nurse practitioners, as well as to encourage third-party payers to be more responsible in helping to support education efforts." Government funding has permitted the private sector to try new approaches to improved delivery, for example, to place nurse practitioner students in group practice or HMO settings," he said. "Without those kinds of monies, we'd be dead."

Service delivery gaps would be equally as crippling if the current combination of training support were to dwindle in the traditional areas of medical education. Proof of the symbiotic relationship that exists between service and training was offered by a spokesman from the Emory University School of Medicine and Grady Memorial Hospital, a teaching affiliate, in Atlanta. He recalled that some years before, several tax commissioners objected to what they considered were exorbitant costs of training at the hospital and hired a major consulting firm to examine whether the hospital was enjoying the same "rich" benefits in the affiliate relationship as was the school. "This firm did an objective study," he reported, "and not only did it find that both institutions were getting a good deal, but also concluded that it would cost the hospital more to contract for the same physician services that were being provided by residents and interns."

"The mutual advantages of this traditional training relationship continue to be overlooked by third-party payers as they seek to avoid supporting clinical training through service reimbursement," another participant added. They must be made aware that the alternatives will cost even more. If current support levels dwindle and eventually disappear, "not only will the universities be left with their tenured professors to support, but the clinical provider of care will be forced to substitute something more expensive for what has been taken away. We're on a collision course," he warned. "Not only will substituting more expensive care result," someone else added, "but also the opportunities for the next generation of practitioners, and hence the next generation of patients to be cared for, which is even more serious, will be limited."

The Drawback of Federal Dollars

Although no one could suggest a feasible way for the medical education system to extricate itself from its dependence on traditional funding sources, especially government sources, workshop participants agreed that those funding relationships had created perhaps as many problems as they had solved. The most visible of these has been the encouragement of fragmentation in medical care through the support of a too narrowly defined host of superspecialties and subspecialties. One participant suggested that "history has to be examined before we make any more recommendations as to what degree of dependence there should be on specialized federal funds for education in medicine." Current high levels of support in cancer and heart research from the National Institutes of Health, for example, are just the most recent category of monies that get funneled into support for specialty training and have caused "the fragmentation of internal medicine into a series of organs."

This kind of educational financing has not only fostered the neglect of primary care, a fault that one participant suggested was being "artificially" corrected through current emphasis on the specialty of family practice, but it has also helped to increase health care costs. "There was a period of about a decade when it was quite easy to get training grants, a large portion of which supported faculty, extra residents, and fellows. Many of those grants are no longer available," one person said, "yet we are now stuck with supporting residents that we would not have if it hadn't been for that federal money in our past." "And eliminating these residencies is nigh onto impossible," another continued, "because they are often the prize of entrenched departmental programs whose chairmen refuse to relinquish any part of their following."

There is certainly something to be said for producing the highly specialized, scrupulously trained physicians that such programs graduate. "On the other hand," someone suggested, "the balance between education and service in a clinical setting that is overstaffed with residents is invariably thrown out of kilter." "I happen to think that most residency programs in academic centers have 30 to 50 percent more residents than they really need to render a service," another person said. "As a result, you get a lot of conferences and seminars to keep people busy because the programs have outgrown their service load." This shift away from the bedside and into the classroom encourages future health care professionals to forget that the patient is in fact the teacher. "Medical specialty boards can in part be faulted for this trend," he continued, "as they define more and more precisely the body of knowledge and the training approach they believe are necessary to produce quality practitioners. The typical teaching hospital with a medical school affiliation offers a range of services to patients that are often dictated by the philosophy of the medical school, which, in turn, is greatly influenced by the philosophy of the specialty boards. Eventually, this influence can be traced to the question of whether we have adequate and appropriate physician manpower in this country," he continued.

Another unfortunate and costly side effect of the dependence of medical schools on federal funding is the uncertainty of annual appropriations, which are usually not made final until after the schools have had to commit themselves to faculty and students. Furthermore, this commitment, unlike the federal one that is limited to yearly periods, is made for four years or so in the case of students with grants and for indefinite longer periods in the case of tenured faculty. When government appropriations do not meet expected levels, the medical schools are left scrambling for the dollars to fill those commitments, and finding those dollars can be more expensive when they must come through current patient service reimbursement mechanisms.

ALTERNATIVE FINANCING ROUTES
Relief from these disadvantages could be won only at the price of losing government funding, an unacceptable solution for almost all institutions of medical education. Most alternatives to the current arrangement seem beset with even more problems. For example, one participant suggested that residents' salaries be paid in part out of fees that physicians receive for patient service performed by residents under their supervision. This could reduce the resident payroll burden for the hospital. However, it might not reduce the total expense to the hospital, one person countered, "because it would not simply be a matter of slicing the pie a little differently. The hospital would in effect be paying on a fee-for-service basis rather than getting as many services as one can squeeze from a resident on a fixed salary."

On the other hand, someone else argued that hospitals now pay a resident's supervisor a full salary for *not* performing the service that the resident performs. Another person suggested that this apparent double payment must be considered in light of another factor. Many hospitals in their relationship with physicians who supervise clinical education have an arrangement by which those physicians perform hands-on patient care "but turn the money that they have earned over to a hospital fund for the betterment of their respective department. If, for example, you have a chief of surgery who spends some time doing surgery, which he naturally must do to maintain his skills, he can earn fees that exceed the amount of his salary, that is, pay his salary plus contribute to the department's fund. This money might be used to hire another doctor who does research to maintain the institution's academic excellence or who participates in the educational program.

"Furthermore," this person continued, "it's not uncommon that the physician who is hired with such extra funds manages the department's clinic and therefore provides care to patients who would otherwise be underserved. Many of us teaching providers get the money from wherever we can without duplicating billing for the same service," he concluded, "and we then go through a reallocation process inside the hospital to put the money where it could do the most good." Asking that physicians directly share their fees with the residents they supervise would destroy this relationship and would deny the hospital the flexibility to use those monies for more useful and appropriate purposes, which develop and change with time.

A final and important drawback of a resident's sharing in the fee of his supervisor is the probable psychological effect on his approach to the patient service he performs. The shared fee might encourage the resident to change his focus from learning to earning, an undesirable attitude at any point in the formal training process.

Another suggestion participants considered for finding alternative means of financing medical education was to readjust third-party reimbursement formulas so that hospitals affiliated with medical schools might be reimbursed at a higher rate than those not involved in education. Third-party payers would "save" money by reimbursing nonteaching institutions at a comparatively lower rate.

However, one participant pointed out that this approach suffers from the same risks as the recommendation, previously discussed, of separating the education from the service component in reimbursement. "One of the mechanisms that is now evolving for determining what might represent reasonable reimbursement in general is a peer group comparison among providers," he continued.

The same approach might eventually be used in differentiating teaching from nonteaching hospitals. However, unless the differentiation was precise, fair reimbursement levels would not be developed because "within the group that does teaching, there are various degrees of education going on with various levels of costs attached."

An added risk of differential reimbursement formulas is that the related differential hospital rates among the various hospitals in any given community would tend to discourage potential patients from agreeing to be admitted to the hospitals with higher rates, for example, the teaching institutions. The long-term effect of such a patient boycott would be staggering.

Despite these drawbacks, a properly developed differential reimbursement formula is a much more attractive alternative to the currently used standard formula, which imposes considerable hardships on teaching hospitals. "I've argued with the health division of the New York Welfare Department," one participant recounted, "that our institutions would be delighted to charge $27 a day for a tonsillectomy if we could get $190 a day, which is what it costs us, to care for a three year old with third-degree burns on 30 percent of the child's body. However, if the department sends us a patient load 85 percent of which is composed of unusually expensive cases and expects us as a teaching institution to be paid a standard rate, then the state, which collects the taxes, must tax Blue Cross subscribers and self-pay patients and the endowment of the hospital something extra to make up the difference in our costs."

FEWER PHYSICIANS, MORE EXTENDERS

"The continued availability of financial support for physician training," someone suggested, "will have a direct influence on the wider utilization and acceptance of various physician extenders, specifically physician's assistants and nurse practitioners." Not only will this be true in inner-city hospitals, especially if primary care physicians are not trained in sufficient numbers, but it will also affect the entire health care industry to some degree. Someone else predicted that there will be an even greater impact if some form of national health insurance is passed, with the resulting and inevitable increased demand for physician services. The available physician manpower will not be able to handle this demand, and so there will be a greater need for physician extenders and allied health care personnel.

Everyone agreed that it is unfortunate, but perhaps not surprising, that physician extenders, who were supposed to be a great boon to such underserved areas as the inner city, have not been employed more widely. The nonstandardized training programs for physician's assistants have been one reason for administrators' and physicians' reluctance to accept this new type of health care practitioner. Another understandable reason for reluctance has been the question of liability for the new practitioners' activities. This is an especially pressing issue in light of the recent furor over rising malpractice insurance premiums. Less understandable has been the refusal of some physicians to relinquish any part of their medical domain to the new professionals. A similar professional rivalry has also been apparent among nurses, who regard the nurse practitioner as not quite one of their own but not a physician either.

Both phenomena continue to stand in the way of achieving innovative and necessary primary care in underserved communities. In some cases, "standing in the way" amounts to downright economic sabotage. One participant recounted the story of an "area of rural Kentucky that was served by only one elderly physician. A clinic operated mainly by physicians' assistants with physician backup was established. The two physicians on the clinic's staff apparently saw this as an economic opportunity, withdrew from the clinic, established their own practice, and began a price competition with the clinic. The physicians were successful in driving the clinic out of existence because the region could not support two systems," he continued. "Once the clinic closed down, the doctors' prices went up."

There is not much that can be done to eliminate this and other more subtle kinds of rivalry between traditional and newer health care professionals. However, participants agreed that greater attention must be paid lest other developments restrict inner-city hospitals' flexibility in using the skills of new health care practitioners. Licensure, for example, has become the goal of many allied health care manpower groups, because they see in it greater economic gain, increased prestige, and the recognition that they are quite capable of working beside the two traditionally licensed groups, physicians and nurses.

The claim that licensure ensures high-quality care makes its implementation for every practitioner group additionally attractive to the public. "However, there is no evidence to support this claim," one person said. "The only way licensure might possibly protect the public is by establishing an entry level." However, there is ample evidence that licensure restricts flexible utilization of allied health care skills. In its present form, then, licensure is an inefficient and therefore costly approach to manpower management. Several participants urged that current attempts to establish some form of national allied health care manpower certification be encouraged to prevent a further multiplication of the ill effects that licensure has caused, especially in underserved and underfinanced areas.

UNION ACTIVITY IN SCARCITY

Similar ill effects can be seen in institutions in which employee unions have operated for some time. "It is going to be impossible for hospitals to respond to new initiatives to take people from one type of job to another," someone said, "to provide employee mobility, to make them more satisfied workers while also filling the hospital's skilled manpower needs, if unions and their negotiating processes protect the status quo in job definitions."

"Another participant suggested that not all union activity is designed to immobilize the system in this way. As a matter of fact, when money is scarce, and the union knows it, its bargaining focus, more often than not, is the betterment of its members' work opportunities through such devices as career mobility. "If unions outside the health care industry can serve as any kind of predictor," he continued, "unions in hospitals under conditions of scarce resources should turn their attention to accepting some responsibility for the health of the industry. If we are talking about shrinking down the system, then the responsible and imaginative union organization will be able to cushion the impact of the shrinkage by seeing that its members can do the jobs that need doing." Responsible unions, in cooperation with enlightened management, should, between them, be able to arrive at workable solutions to fill hospital's manpower needs.

SYMPATHETIC BUT TOUGH

Responsibility, enlightened conduct, cooperativeness, rationality—these qualities were important to participants no matter which end of the health care manpower spectrum they were discussing, from unskilled workers represented by unions through allied health care groups to physician specialists. The opinions they expressed on manpower issues demonstrated a sympathy for and an understanding of each group's seeking the most profitable and satisfying work environment.

Nevertheless, the participants clearly implied that moderation would have to govern all future manpower activity if the needs of the underserved were to be met to even a minimal degree. They agreed that urban health care institutions could no longer sustain the inflationary pressures of too many superspecialists and not enough primary care practitioners, of multiplying allied health care groups seeking parity with the traditional professions, and of costly and restrictive union demands. If the financial resources at the health care system's disposal continue to shrink, then everyone, the institutions as well as the individuals who work in them, will have to exercise control in balancing their demands with the needs of the patients whom they intend to serve.

Reference
1. Medenhall, R. C., and others. A national study of medical and surgical specialties. III. An empirical approach to the classification of patient care. *J. Amer. Assn.* 241:2180-85, May 18, 1979.

Summary and Recommendations

Some Familiar Exhortations

If there is one message that can summarize the conference deliberations and generally describe the multitude of problems that all health care institutions must deal with, it is simply that the current organization of health care delivery does not make sense. The often-heard complaint that there is no system to the system continues to be true. It is not surprising, then, that all the conference recommendations, individually and as a whole, represent a call for rationality.

Doubtless the most rational of these recommendations is a response to the not-infrequent question heard throughout the conference: should solutions be developed within the framework of traditional health care institutions, or should the whole system be scrapped and begun again from scratch? The response, of course, is that neither extreme will do. The former suggestion has already been tried with only limited success, and the latter, while a good indicator of the frustration that plagues the system's many would-be reformers, is just not feasible. In fact, a hasty surrender to such frustration may have been the cause of many of the problems conference participants gathered to discuss.

For example, the widespread fragmentation among delivery programs as well as in manpower training has been caused in part by federal funding for projects being withdrawn too quickly because of impatience with results that were slow in coming. The same sort of urge for fast solutions, although understandable in light of the drastic needs of the underserved, continues to encourage neglect of well-designed research in health care delivery. As a result, even the value of those research projects that have been mounted has too often been lost for want of careful evaluation and dissemination of results.

Another major drawback of haste in problem solving and of communities' eagerness to embrace any and all outside help has been the imposition of federal solutions on local problems. Complaints about the inappropriateness of federally administered programs implemented at the local level were frequently voiced during the conference as participants searched for ways to increase federal dollars without simultaneously having to submit to inflexible and often contradictory federal regulations. Considering the financial plight of urban centers, most participants reluctantly agreed that you cannot have one without at least a smattering of the other.

As one participant put it, "If we're going to ask the federal government to take immediate steps to provide financial relief for health care facilities that serve large numbers of unsponsored and poor patients, we must expect to give something in return. It's not unreasonable for the government to ask the cities to restructure local health care programs so they more realistically meet the needs of this large population group in a more efficient and cost-effective manner. Too many of us have been too long preoccupied with the idea that national health insurance would be the ultimate answer to all of our problems," he continued. In the meantime, very little has been done to address the specific problems that face urban underserved areas. "Perhaps we ought to spend a little less time philosophizing about national health insurance," he concluded, "and begin to tackle very aggressively the problems of financing and organizing health care for the very large populations of underserved in urban areas."

PAYMENT FOR HEALTH CARE
The conference's recommendations on payment for health care fell into three interrelated areas: financing, planning and organization, and manpower. The fact that none of the recommendations presents an earthshaking discovery or a newfound wisdom indicates that the problems are long-standing ones and that the possible solutions have not been applied to a sufficient degree to take hold and make a long-term, significant improvement. Only the extent of the need has changed. Conference discussions were replete with stories of service cutbacks, lower reimbursements, and reduced eligibility for coverage among the urban poor. The one increase anyone could point to was in numbers of patients who applied for care but could not demonstrate having financial support from any source.

Increased financing, then, is one major area of concern to urban health care institutions. As one participant described the situation, "All of our major cities face severe fiscal problems, and in the majority of them, the costs of providing health care services have increased as rapidly as, if not more rapidly than, all other costs involved in operating urban municipalities. Local tax resources have become so limited that unless increased fiscal support for health care is forthcoming from other areas, that is, state and federal governments, services will have to be reduced rather significantly in the future."

Summary and Recommendations 99

The message that conference participants made very clear echoed the conclusions of the Commission on Public-General Hospitals report that money for urban health care institutions must be found, it must be found immediately, and the most likely source is the federal government.[1] However, unlike much past federal support, future monies must be disbursed in a more rational way—"an infusion of federal funds creatively utilized," one person called it.

Specifically, the following recommendations were made:
- The piecemeal approach of past federal funding that encourages fragmentation and disarticulation of services must be avoided.
- When short-term programs are initiated, they must be maintained until local financing can undertake their continued support.
- Existing grant demonstration or experimental programs should be used to selectively channel funds to improve basic services as well as to encourage new delivery programs.
- Health care delivery programs to targeted groups of poor must be initiated more widely, with emphasis on developing primary care and on increasing support for existing and new community health care centers whose programs are coordinated with those of hospitals and other health care or social service agencies.
- Attempts must be made to eliminate overutilization of some federally supported programs by changing reimbursement regulations that encourage inappropriate care.
- Fiscal assistance must be provided to urban hospitals to help them meet current fire-safety and life-safety codes and licensure requirements, but only within the general guidelines of health care planning for a given service area.
- Reimbursement levels must reflect hospital's financial requirements and so provide for the servicing of debt and the replenishment of capital. Toward this end, Medicaid reimbursement formulas should be equalized across all participating states.
- A more creative approach embodying appropriate incentives is required, not just to attract, but also to retain increasing numbers of health care professionals in the urban setting. Among these incentives should be improvement of the physical environment in which health care professionals work and an assurance that their services would be rewarded with reasonably competitive compensation.
- Where possible, the expansion of the fee-for-service compensation approach to new groups of health care professionals should be regarded as inflationary and therefore should be discouraged.
- Existing financial incentives for reorganizing health care services should be maintained, and new and promising incentives should

be sought and implemented. For example, if the Medicaid waiver authority were broadened, the potential for developing health maintenance organization (HMO) prototypes in underserved areas could be significantly increased. Furthermore, development and start-up capital should be available to stimulate the growth of such provider units in the inner city. Toward this end, Congress should be encouraged to support experimentation and permit health care providers to engage in some massive, long-term capitation arrangements with low-income populations without having to submit to the criteria that govern entrepreneurial HMOs.
- If possible, existing financing mechanisms for service reimbursement should be relied upon to assist communities in financing the debt of hospitals that are obsolete and/or necessary. Regulations that govern debt management should be made more flexible.

DELIVERY OF HEALTH CARE

To ensure the efficient and creative use of such monies as will be made available to improve urban health care, conference participants recommended some basic changes in the organization of services:
- All hospitals in a given area—private as well as public, inner city as well as suburban—should cooperate in the reorganization effort and submit equally to planning regulations.
- Although federal standards are necessary to ensure high quality, regulations governing the use of various program funds should be flexible enough to permit each health care delivery area to organize and use those funds in a manner appropriate to its unique situation.
- The hospital should remain the most appropriate focus for coordinating all health care services in the community. Nevertheless, dispersed facilities for communities underserved in primary care should be made available where they are appropriate.
- Changes in Medicaid regulations permitting the development of organized ambulatory and comprehensive care programs for pre-enrolled populations should be encouraged. These programs would be funded on a capitation basis.
- The mechanisms of merger and consolidation should be used whenever possible to eliminate unnecessary hospital facilities. Where appropriate, such facilities could also be converted to other health care or social service uses.
- To relieve urban hospitals of the burden and cost of caring for patients with nonmedical problems who often have no other

source of help, municipalities must begin to operate 24-hour, seven-day-a-week social service agencies. Furthermore, each urban area should have a single agency that coordinates services for individuals with multiple problems. This agency must have access to both public and private sources of service.
- Informal social service systems should be encouraged so that communities might better help themselves by promoting early intervention in incipient problems among members and so helping to prevent some crisis situations.
- To ensure continuity of care and avoid costly duplication of services to individuals who use multiple provider sources, each patient's complete medical record should be automatically available to and used by every provider who is responsible for some aspect of the patient's health care. Where possible, exchange of patient information among providers could be encouraged by tying it to the reimbursement mechanism.

CONSUMER POWER AND MEDICAL MANPOWER
This last set of recommendations, as well as all the preceding ones, is intended to foster what must be the health care system's ideal situation: continuity of care, which is another way of saying rational health care services. If the system is to achieve this goal for every patient, four essential components must be put into place: an integrated, comprehensive health care benefits package; an organized delivery system that links all sources of care; a primary care physician who accepts responsibility for planning and coordinating all the health care needs of a patient and family; and an informed patient whose complete health record follows him to every new provider of care.

Conference participants emphasized the importance of the last two components and recognized the sorry lack of both, despite some recent strides in primary care training and consumer health education. "Both provider and patient have to become disciples of the philosophy of continuity of care," one participant said. To fill this gap, the conference recommended the following:
- Current patient education efforts must be continued and expanded, and new programs that attract and benefit the community must be developed.
- Patient education should be designed so that specific patient populations are instructed in how to comply with therapeutic regimens and so that the community is encouraged to adopt life-styles that are healthier, to practice maintaining good health, and to develop informal networks for self-help.

- Because a successful self-help network depends on community members' being informed about all available health care and social service resources, health care institutions and such units as the local Health Systems Agency must inform the community about their activities and in turn seek the community's input.
- Despite their initial ignorance about the complexities of health care delivery, consumers' input should be included either formally or informally in the various goal-setting and decision-making processes of health care institutions and agencies.

Conference participants agreed that just as the hospital is likely to remain the focus of a community's health care services, the physician will continue to be the care giver with the primary responsibility for managing a patient's therapy, at least for the foreseeable future. However, they noted that the current generation of physicians does not include a sufficient proportion of primary care or family practitioners nor are they distributed well throughout the system. The solutions to this combination of shortage and maldistribution may be expected from implementation of the following recommendations:

- Medical schools in urban underserved areas and major medical centers must cooperate and assume the responsibility for developing programs that attract students and practitioners to primary care in the inner city. If such a voluntary approach is not effective, federally mandated distribution and federally sponsored physician-supply programs must be seriously considered as alternatives.
- Both the physical and the practical environments of inner-city health care facilities must be made more attractive, not only to better recruit more practitioners, but also to foster a genuine commitment among those who currently work there.
- Medical schools must make a special effort to develop among their faculty members family practice role models who are as appealing to students as the role models they find in other specialties. This may entail establishing a special tenure track for such faculty members, who do not often have extensive experience in academic settings.
- In cooperation with inner-city hospitals and/or other primary care provider units, the medical school must ensure that its family practice residents are provided with relevant experience in primary care practice environments.
- Family practice curriculums must be refined to better reflect patient's primary care needs and to more effectively develop students' expertise and sense of responsibility through longer rotations specifically designed for primary care training.

- Generally, the medical school in the urban environment must consciously develop a philosophy of service to its immediate community and carefully recruit faculty and students who will embody that commitment in practice.
- To ensure that training programs produce greater numbers of family practitioners, a better balance must be found in the financing of various categories of medical training. Emphasis on funding narrowly defined specialty training must be abondoned in favor of supporting medical education that produces the kinds and the numbers of practitioners that will fill the population's needs.
- Third-party payers must be strongly encouraged to maintain the traditional tie between financing training and reimbursing for services, whether the students be in medicine or in any of the related health care professions.
- To complement physician primary care in underserved areas, utilization of physician extenders and other health care professionals must be encouraged, and attention must be given to preventing rigid licensure and accreditation developments that decrease the system's flexibility and efficiency in using health care manpower skills.

PUTTING IT ALL TOGETHER

One participant noted that these recommendations are all based on "some pretty safe beliefs." However, the probability of any of them becoming reality is not at all a safe wager because they all depend on an increase in two scarce commodities: money and a cooperation that grows out of a rational approach to the complex problems of the system. Not only must understanding of the intricate relationship of needs and resources be fostered within the system, among its decision makers and administrators and health care professionals, but also the force of rationality must be brought to bear on the deliberations and decisions of state and federal governments.

To emphasize that success depends on this kind of enlightenment, participants developed three final recommendations that describe the most promising scheme for alleviating the plight of health care institutions in the inner city:

- *Cooperation among public and private institutions.* In order to make good their claim that the design of health care services is much better accomplished at the local level, public and private institutions in the inner city must cooperate with one another to develop complementary services rather than compete for already scarce resources.

- *New program funding based on careful research.* The development of new, more effective delivery methods to the urban underserved must rely on a careful evaluation of needs, on the results of successful experimental projects conducted elsewhere, and on the meticulous forecasting of probable costs. There are no available data describing the current cost of financing the health care that presently exists in underserved urban areas. Research in this field must be conducted as soon as possible so that proposals for increased service may be presented with cost estimates that are creditable to both legislatures and the taxpaying public.
- *United effort to make health for all a national priority.* There must be a shift in the approach of the many and disparate health-related groups that apply to legislatures for assistance. Armed with the kind of information that careful research and experience can provide, health care organizations must present a united front in convincing the public and its representatives that maintaining the nation's health must become a national priority and that resources lavished elsewhere must be redirected toward caring for the poor and underserved.

Reference
1. Hospital Research and Educational Trust. *The Future of the Public-General Hospital: An Agenda for Transition.* Chicago: HRET, 1978.

Selected Bibliography

General

Bennett, B., and Norman, J. C., editors. *Medicine in the Ghetto.* New York City: Appleton-Century-Crofts, 1969.

Blendon, R. J. The reform of ambulatory care: a financial paradox. *Med. Care.* 14:526, June 1976.

Cantor, M., and Mayer, M. Health and the inner city elderly, part 1. *The Gerontologist.* 16:17, Feb. 1976.

Carp, F. M., and Kataoka, E. Health care problems of the elderly of San Francisco's Chinatown, part 1. *The Gerontologist.* 16:30, Feb. 1976.

Cervantes, R. A. The failure of comprehensive health services to serve the urban Chicano. *Health Serv. Rep.* 87:932, Dec. 1972.

Couto, R. A. Poverty, politics, and health care: an Appalachian experience. New York City: Praeger Publishers, 1975.

Eddins, E. A. Proposed changes in health care practices in the black community. *Amer. J. Orthopsychiatry.* 42:222, Mar. 1972.

Elling, R. H., and Martin, R. F. *Health and Health Care for the Urban Poor* (Connecticut Health Services Research Series no. 5). North Haven, CT: 1974.

German, P. S., and others. Ambulatory care for chronic conditions in an inner-city elderly population. *Amer. J. Public Health.* 66:660, July 1976.

Ginsberg, E. *Urban Health Services: The Case of New York City.* New York City: Columbia University Press, 1971.

Hammonds, K. E. Blacks and the urban health crisis. *J. Nat. Med. Assn.* 66:226, May 1974.

King, W. M. Health, health care and the black community: an exploratory bibliography. Monticello, IL: The Council, 1974.

Komaroff, A. L., and Duffell, P. J. An evaluation of selected federal categorical health programs for the poor. *Amer. J. Public Health.* 66:255, Mar. 1976.

Miller, C. A. Health care of children and youth in America. *Amer. J. Public Health.* 65:353, Apr. 1975.

Milt, H., editor. *Health Care Problems of the Inner City.* New York City: National Health Council, 1969.

Newberger, E. H., and others. Child health in America: toward a rational public policy. *Milbank Memorial Fund Quarterly.* 54:249, Summer 1976.

Porter, P. J., and others. Municipal child health services: a ten-year reorganization—Cambridge, MA. *Pediat.* 58:704, Nov. 1976.

Roghmann, K. J. Looking for the medical care crisis in utilization data. *Inquiry, Blue Cross Association.* 11:282, Dec. 1974.

Seham, M. *Blacks and American Medical Care.* Minneapolis: University of Minnesota Press, 1973.

Thompson, T., and Hicks, F. J., editors. *Health Policy and Planning in the Urban Community.* Silver Spring, MD: Ebon Research Systems, 1975.

Tierney, J. T., and Morton, M., editor. *Sickness and Poverty.* Washington: Community Health Service, U.S. Government Printing Office, 1971.

Weiss, J. H., and Leveson, I., editors. *Analysis of Urban Health Problems.* New York City: Halsted Press, 1976.

White, E. H. Health and the black person: an annotated bibliography. *Amer. J. Nurs.* 74:1839, Oct. 1974.

Urban Resources

Bergen Jr., S. S., and Schatzki, M. New directions for an urban hospital: Fort Green, New York City. *J. Amer. Med. Assn.* 215:935, Feb. 1971.

Boyajian, L. Z. History strikes again: two 20th-century reform ventures. *Hosp. Community Psych.* 26:17, Jan. 1975.

Brook, R. H., and Williams, K. N. Quality of health care for the disadvantaged. *J. Community Health.* 1:132, Winter 1975.

Brunswick, A. F. Indicators of health status in adolescence. *Int. J. Health Services.* 6:475, 1976.

Challenor, B. D., and others. Community medicine: an evolving discipline. *Ann. Intern. Med.* 76:689, May 1972.

Coe, R. M., and others. Impact of Medicare on the organization of community health resources. *Milbank Memorial Fund Quarterly.* 52:231, Summer 1974.

Haughton, J. G. The role of the public-general hospital in community health. *Amer. J. Public Health.* 65:21, Jan. 1975.

Health care in St. Louis, parts 1 and 2. *Urban Health.* 6:16, Mar. 1977; 6:34, Apr. 1977.

Johnson, T. M., and Stein, G. H. Politics and personality in medicine: genesis of an indigent clinic. *Amer. J. Public Health.* 65:253, Mar. 1975.

Mann Jr., J. B. Black community's crisis of care hits hospitals and consumers. *Hospitals, J.A.H.A.* 51:70, Mar. 16, 1977.

McKinney, E. A. Health care crisis—for whom? *Health and Social Work.* 1:101, Feb. 1976.

Merten, W., and Nothman, S. Neighborhood health center experience: implications for project grants. *Amer. J. Public Health.* 65:243, Mar. 1975.

Novack, A. H., and others. Children's mental health services in an inner city neighborhood: 3-year epidemiological study. *Amer. J. Public Health.* 65:133, Feb. 1975.

Piore, N., and others. *Health Expenditures in New York City: A Decade of Change.* New York City: Columbia University Center for Community Health Systems, 1976.

Porter, P. J., and others. Municipal child health services: ten-year reorganization—Cambridge, MA. *Pediat.* 58:704, Nov. 1976.

Primary Care Development Project. *Prescription for Primary Health Care: A Community Guidebook.* Ithaca, NY: Cornell University, 1976.

Rosenberger, D. M. The urban hospital system. *J. Amer. College Hosp. Admin.* 17:18, Summer 1972.

Schacter, L. P., and Elliston, E. P. Medical care in a free community clinic. *J. Amer. Med. Assn.* 237:1848, Apr. 25, 1977.

Straker, N., and others. The use of two-way TV in bringing mental health services to the inner city: East Harlem. *Amer. J. Psych.* 133:1202, Oct. 1976.

Taietz, P. Community complexity and knowledge of facilities. *J. Gerontology.* 30:357, 1975.

Warnecke, R. B., and others. Contact with health guides and use of health services among blacks in Buffalo. *Public Health Rep.* 90:213, May-June 1975.

Waybur, A. *Analysis of Diverse Modes of Organization for Medical Care of the Poor.* Los Angeles: University of California, 1974.

Weinstein, B. M. Bellevue opts for modernization by renovating physical facilities and realigning administrative functions. *Hospitals, J.A.H.A.* 47:44, Nov. 1973.

Weinstein, B. M., and Lesser, D. Health manpower: annual administrative review. *Hospitals, J.A.H.A.* 48:67, Apr. 1974.

Accessibility and Acceptability of Health Services

Aday, L. A. The impact of health policy on access to medical care. *Milbank Memorial Fund Quarterly.* 54:215, Spring 1976.

Alpert, J. J., and others. Delivery of health care for children: report of an experiment. *Pediat.* 57:917, June 1976.

Bergen, S. S., and Schatzki, M. New directions for an urban hospital: Fort Green, New York City. *J. Amer. Med. Assn.* 215:935, Feb. 8, 1971.

Bullough, B., and Bullough, V. L. *Poverty, Ethnic Identity, and Health Care.* New York City: Appleton-Century-Crofts, 1972.

Coleman, A. H. A social system to improve health care delivery to the poor: San Francisco. *J. Nat. Med. Assn.* 61:192, Mar. 1969.

Detwiller, L. F. The right to health. *Hospitals, J.A.H.A.* 45:63, Feb. 16, 1971.

Douglass, C. W. Consumer influence in health planning in the urban ghetto. *Inquiry, Blue Cross Association.* 12:157, June 1975.

Dummett, C. O. Consumer-provider conflict in health service recommendations. *Health Serv. Rep.* 88:795, Nov. 1973.

Falkson, J. L. An evaluation of alternative models of citizen participation in urban bureaucracy. Ann Arbor: Program in Health Planning, School of Public Health, University of Michigan, 1971.

Fried, C. An analysis of equality and rights in medical care. *Hosp. Progr.* 57:44, Feb. 1976.

Gottlieb, S. R. Data requirements for areawide health planning agencies. *Med. Care.* 8:175, July-Aug. 1970.

Green, L. W., and others. Research and demonstration issues in self-care: measuring the decline of medicocentrism. *Health Educ. Monographs.* 5:161, Summer 1977.

Gross, P. F. Urban health disorders, spatial analysis, and the economics of health facility location. *Int. J. Health Serv.* 2:63, Feb. 1972.

Hertz, P., and Stamps, P. L. Appointment-keeping behavior re-evaluated. *Amer. J. Public Health.* 67:1033, Nov. 1977.

Hiscock, W. M. Urban and regional foundations for health planning. *Public Health Rep.* 85:267, Mar. 1970.

Hospital Research and Educational Trust. *The Contemporary Status of Large Urban Public Hospitals—Ambulatory Services.* Summary Report of the Large Urban Public Hospitals Ambulatory Services Project. School of Public Health, University of California, Los Angeles. Chicago: HRET, 1972.

Kaplan, R. S., and Leinhardt, S. The spatial distribution of urban pharmacies. *Med. Care.* 13:37, Jan. 1975.

Lewis, H. L. A pioneering diocesan hospital system—10-year status report Catholic Medical Center of Brooklyn & Queens, Inc. *Hosp. Progr.* 58:60, Jan.-June 1977.

McNamara, J. J. Communities and control of health services. *Inquiry, Blue Cross Association.* 9:64, Sept. 1972.

Milio, N. Self-care in urban settings. *Health Educ. Monographs.* 5:136, Summer 1977.

Okada, L. M., and Sparer, G. Access to usual source of care by race and income in ten urban areas. *J. Community Health.* 1:163, Spring 1976.

Piore, N. Who delivers primary care? *Bull. New York Acad. Med.* 53:124, Jan.-Feb. 1977.

Quesada, G. M., and Heller, P. L. Sociocultural barriers to medical care among Mexican-Americans in Texas: a summary report of research conducted by the Southwest Medical Sociology Ad Hoc Committee. *Med. Care.* 15:93, May 1977.

Rice, H. To cure racism. *Hospitals, J.A.H.A.* 47:54, May 1, 1973.

Russell, M. V. Social work in a black community hospital: its implications for the profession—Harlem Hospital, New York City. *Amer. J. Public Health.* 60:704, Apr. 1970.

Salkever, D. S. Economic class and differential access to care: comparisons among health care systems. *Int. J. Health Serv.* 5:373, 1975.

Salkever, D. S. and others. Episodes of illness and access to care in the inner city: a comparison of HMO and non-HMO populations. *Health Serv. Res.* 11:252, Feb. 1976.

Satcher, D., and others. Family practice for the inner city: what consumers expect. *Urban Health.* 5:36, Oct. 1976.

Smith, D. B., and Kaluzny, A. D. Inequality in health care programs: a note on some structural factors affecting health care behavior. *Med. Care.* 12:860, Oct. 1974.

Wang, V. L., and others. An approach to consumer-patient activation in health maintenance—a report of the Maryland 1-year health education demonstration project. *Public Health Rep.* 90:449, Sept.-Oct. 1975.

Manpower

Bergen Jr., S. S. Physician manpower: the issues. *J. Med. Soc. New Jersey.* 70:557, Aug. 1973.

Public hospital: a suitable teaching resource? *Hosp. Med. Staff.* 2:23, May 1973.

Daugirdas, J. T. The urban doctors program: Northwestern University Medical School. *J. Amer. Med. Assn.* 218:1197, Nov. 22, 1971.

Fenninger, L. D. Health services in the USA: trends in the education and training of health personnel. *World Health Organization Public Health Paper.* (60):26, 1974.

_____. Health manpower and the education of health personnel. *Inquiry, Blue Cross Association.* 10:56-60+, Mar. 1973 (Pt 2).

Ginsberg, E., and Yokalem, A. M., editors. University Medical Center and the Metropolis. Paper from the Conference on the Medical Center and the Metropolis, Columbia University, 1973. New York City: Josiah Macy Jr. Foundation, 1974.

Hirschfeld, A. H. Medicine in the inner city. *Delaware Med. J.* 42:57, Mar. 1970.

Institute of Labor and Industrial Relations. *Poverty and Human Resources Abstracts.* Beverly Hills, CA: Sage Press, no date.

_____. *Poverty and Human Resources Abstracts.* Beverly Hills, CA: Sage Press, no date.

Lee, F. E., and Glasser, J. H. Role of lay midwifery in maternity care in a large metropolitan area. *Public Health Rep.* 89:537, Nov.-Dec., 1974.

Paxton, G. S., and others. A core city problem: recruitment and retention of salaried physicians. *Med. Care.* 13:209, Mar. 1975.

Public hospital: a suitable teaching resource? *Hosp. Med. Staff.* 2:23, May 1973.